Avicenna On the Breath

Adapted By

Laleh Bakhtiar

From Translations by
O. Cameron Gruner and Mazar H. Shah
Correlated with the Arabic by Jay R. Crook
with Notes by O. Cameron Gruner

Great Books of the Islamic World, Inc.

Printed in the United States of America.

Library of Congress Cataloging-in-Publication Data

Ibn Sina, Abu Ali al-Husayn ibn Abd Allah
The Canon of Medicine (al-Qanun fi'l tibb)
Lecture 7 - On the Breath
1. Islam. 2. Medicine. I. Title

ISBN 10 (Book): 1-56744-998-0
ISBN 13 (Book): 978-1-56744-998-3
ISBN 10 (eBook): 1-56744-999-9
ISBN 13 (eBook): 978-1-56744-999-0

Cover Design by Liaquat Ali
Cornerstones are Allah and Muhammad connected by Bismillah al-Rahman al-Rahim (In the Name of God, the Merciful, the Compassionate).

Design and layout by Abir Usman

Published by
Great Books of the Islamic World, Inc.

Distributed by
KAZI Publications, Inc.
3023 W. Belmont Avenue
Chicago IL 60618
Tel: 773-267-7001; FAX: 773-267-7002
email: info@kazi.org

Contents

Endnotes

Introduction by Laleh Bakhtiar

In the Name of God, the Merciful, the Compassionate

I. Biographical Sketch

The "Prince of Physicians," Abu Al Sina (Avicenna) (b. 370/980) was born in Afshana. By the age of ten he had learned the entire Quran as well as grammar and then began the study of logic and mathematics. Once these subjects were mastered, he studied physics, metaphysics and medicine. By the age of sixteen he had mastered all of the sciences of his day except metaphysics. While he had read Aristotle's Metaphysics over and over again and had even memorized it, he could not understand it until he read al-Farabi's commentary on it. Avicenna was then eighteen years old.

He was favored by the ruler of Bukhara because of his mastery of medicine, but when he was thirty-two, he was forced to migrate because of the political situation in his home town area. He migrated to Jurjan on the southeast coast of the Caspian Sea in an attempt to join the court of the well-known Qabus ibn Wushmgir. This never materialized as the ruler had died in 1013 during Avicenna's travels to Jurjan. Avicenna then retired to a village near Jurjan where he was to meet his disciple-to-be, al-Juzjani.

Al-Juzjani was devoted to Avicenna and was to write commentaries upon his works as well as to preserve copies of all of the master's writings. It was in Jurjan in 1012 that Avicenna wrote the beginning of his great medical text, *The Canon (al-Qanun)* on medicine. Avicenna remained in Jurjan for two or three years before moving to Rey in 405/1014 or 406/1015, a city near present day Tehran and from there to Hamadan in the northwest Iran. He became a minister in the Buyuid Court of Shams al-Dawlah as well as the court physician. Once again Avicenna was obliged to migrate because of the unstable political conditions in Hamadan so he moved to Isfahan where he enjoyed a fifteen year period of peace, writing many of his major works at that time.

Eventually, however, he was forced to migrate once again and moved back to Hamadan where he died in 428/1037.

II. Avicennian Corpus

One of the leading scholars on Avicenna and the editor of this series, Seyyed Hossein Nasr, has written the following:

> The writings of Avicenna, of which nearly 250 have survived, if we take all his short treatises and letters into account, range over nearly every subject known to the medieval world. These works are mostly in Arabic, but occasionally in Persian, as for example, the *Danish namah-i ala* (The Book of Science Dedicated to Ala al-Dawlah), which is the first philosophic work in modern Persian. Avicenna's Arabic style in his earlier works is rather difficult and uneven; and it was only during his long sojourn in Isfahan-when under the criticism of certain literary experts, he began to study Arabic literature intensely-that his style became polished and perfected. The works written later in life, especially the *Isharat wa'l tanbihat*, testify to this change.
>
> Aviennna's philosophical works include his Peripatetic masterpiece *al-Shifa* (The Book of the Remedy), the Latin *Sufficientia*, which is the longest encyclopedia of knowledge ever written by one man, his Najat (The Book of Deliverance), which is a summary of the *Shifa, Uyun al-hikmah* (Fountains of Wisdom), and his last and perhaps greatest masterpiece *Isharat wa 'l-tanbihat* (The Book of Directives and remarks). In addition he wrote a large number of treatises on logic, psychology, cosmology, and metaphysics. There are also the "esoteric" works pertaining to his "Oriental Philosophy" of which the *Risalah fi'l ishq* (Treatise on Love), the Trilogy *Hayy ibn Yaqan* (The Living Son of the Awake), *Risalat al-Tair* (Treatise of the Bird) and Salaman wa Absal, the last three chapters of the *Isharat*, and *Mantiq al-mashriqiyin* (The Logic of the Orientals), which is a part of a larger work now lost, are the most important.
>
> In the sciences, also, Avicenna composed many small treatises dealing with particular problems in physics, meteorology, and so on, as well as sections contained in the larger compendia, especially the *Shifa*, in which is found the most complete exposition of his views on zoology, botany, and geology, as well as psychology, which in Peripatetic philosophy—and contrary to the view of the later schools like the *Ishraqiyyun* is considered as a branch of physics or natural philosophy. As for medicine, Avicenna composed the famous *Qanun*, or *Canon*, which is perhaps the most influential single work in the history of medicine and is still taught in the East today, the *Urjuzah fi'l-tibb* (Poem on Medicine), containing the principles of Islamic medicine in rhyming verses easy to memorize, and a large number of treatises in both Arabic and Persian on various diseases and drugs.
>
> In addition to his philosophical and scientific works, Avicenna wrote several poems in Arabic and Persian of which *Qasidat al-ainiyah* (Ode on the Soul) is deservedly the most famous. Moreover, he wrote several religious works which include not only treatises on particular religious subjects, such as the meaning of fate and free will, but also commentaries upon several chapters of the Quran.

This latter category is particularly important because it was primarily in these commentaries that Avicenna sought to harmonize reason and revelation along lines already begun by *al-Kindi, al-Farabi* and the *Ikhwan al-safa*, continued after him by *Suhrawardi*, and finally brought to its fruition by *Mir Damad* and *Mulla Sadra*. These writings add an important dimension to the already multidimensional corpus of Avicenna's literary output and emphasize the richness of a collection of writings which range from observational and even experimental science to ontology, from mathematics to gnosis and metaphysics, and from logic to commentaries upon the Sacred Book.[1]

III. The Theory and Practice of Islamic Medicine

The traditional concept of medicine[2] differs profoundly from the view held in the modern world because in the traditional view, the spaces —meridians, channels—within the body and what flows through them are of more significance in causing illness than the shapes or organs, members themselves. That is, the emphasis is on that which flows through the channels as the "place" of the soul.

A clear parallel can be seen in traditional Islamic architecture where space is considered to be one of the most direct symbols of Being and it is primordial, all-pervading and, in Islamic cosmology, the locus of the Universal Soul. Space is also structured. Whether one is referring to the macrocosm or the microcosm, they each contain three divisions: body, soul and spirit.

Traditional man tends towards a mode of comprehension which provides a metaphysical interpretation of life, an interpretation that precedes and goes beyond all external perception. This mode of comprehension, or initial interpretation, affects all of man's perceptions because it begins by situating him in the universe. Initially this interpretation determines his awareness of cosmic space as an externalization of the macrocosmic creation which is analogous to his own microcosmic self. This traditional Hermetic concept forms part of the world view incorporated into the Islamic perspective, a view in which the universe is composed of a macrocosm and microcosm, each containing three great divisions: the body (*jism*), the soul (*nafs*) and the spirit (*ruh*).[3]

Depending on one's perspective, one is either drawn from the body through the soul to the Divine Spirit in the external world or from the body inward through the soul to the Hidden Treasure or Divine Spirit within.

Two interpretations of this concept arise which, although apparently different, are essentially the same. In the first, God as Manifest (*al-Zahir*), is the reality of universal externalization. From within the concentric circles of the macrocosm, there is an outward movement from the earth as corporeal manifestation through an all-pervading soul to the enveloping heavens, viewed as the seat of the Divine Spirit. In the second, complementary view of God as Hidden (*al-Batin*), there is an inward movement within the microcosm of man, beginning with his physical presence and moving towards his spiritual center, the Hidden Treasure. The two schemes correspond to each other, at the same time that one is the reverse of the other.[4]

In this structured space, the human being knows where he or she is. Direction is meaningful.

> It is only with reference to the heavens that the apparent indefiniteness of space can be given direction. In this way space acquires a qualitative aspect. The order of the spheres and the movements through the six directions of north, south, east, west, up and down constitute the primary coordinate system within which all creation is situated. All traditional sciences share this common frame of reference.[5]

The concept of place (*makan*) follows a meaningful direction or orientation. A sense of place consists of both a container (*jism*, body) and the contained (soul, spirit, breath).

> [The concept of place] does not have a tangible existence, but exists in the consciousness of the beholder who visually perceives physical boundaries while his intellect perceives [the soul] and spirit as 'contained,' defined within the boundaries.[6]

Within this structured, oriented concept of space as the place of the soul, all of creation contains both active and passive possibilities. The idea of time in motion arises from the active aspect of space while seen in its passive aspect, it is manifested in matter or form which is directly a product of this movement. This concept—that the soul (space) and not the body (shape) should lead in the healing art—is central to an understanding of traditional medicine.

> The esoteric theory of causation describes this motion as the movement of the soul towards the Divine Spirit through space. Thus the locus of time and form is space, which simultaneously manifests its active and passive aspects through motion.[7]

This perspective is the basis for traditional medicine which looks for the simultaneous movement systems which create a continuous flow based on number—three main faculties, three major organs, three souls, four elements, four humours, nine temperaments, and which interact in space, the place of the soul, with the organs, tissues, membranes, etc.

Finally, we come to the concept of rhythm in time which is best described in terms of traditional music based upon the poem with which Jalal al-Din Rum begins his masterful *Mathnawi*.

Hearken to this Reed forlorn,
Breathing, even since twas torn
From its rushy bed, a strain
Of impassioned love and pain.

The Secret of my song, though near,
None can see and none can hear.
Oh, for a friend to know the sign
And mingle all his soul with mine!

'Tis the flame of Love that fired me.
'Tis the wine of Love inspired me.
Wouldst thou learn how lovers bleed.
Hearken, hearken to the Reed![8]

The continuity and harmony of music is well appreciated and may serve to elucidate another aspect of the spiritual meaning of time-form continuity. The reed, in Jalal al-Din Rumi's poem, contains the bifold characteristics of place. Physically, the reed exhibits a *zahir* or external form which is passive to its hollow interior or *batin*, wherein lies the active spirit of the instrument. The music of the reed is symbolically seen as the externalization of an interior movement, just as musical tones work through wind instruments from the inside out. He who hears the music is aware of the inner space and the harmonious encounter of its motion with its outer shell. This interaction, in the traditional view, represents a spiritual synthesis which regards the reed's *zahir* as the body and its *batin* as the spirit, which, through the music of the soul, yearns to return to the reed bed from whence it was plucked, must as man yearns to return to the One from whom he was issued.[9]

The concept of motion associated with the creation of time and space is explored also by Ibn Arabi in his discourses on initial creation and the subsequent manifestations, viewed as the 'Breath of the Compassionate.' Here 'the universe is annihilated at every moment and re-created at the next without there being a temporal separation between the two phases. It returns back to the Divine Essence at every moment while in the phase of contraction and is re-manifested and externalized in that of expansion. . . Creation is renewed at every instant and its apparent 'horizontal' continuity is pierced by the 'Vertical Cause' which integrates every moment of existence into its transcendent Origin.'[10]

Because of the concentration of traditional Islamic medicine on what flows through the inner spaces, it becomes a dynamic system. That is, the whole is present and operative in each individual locus in which each individual locus knows, so to speak, its position in the whole, its relation to center. The dynamic qualities of the elements can be understood as manifestations of an orderly action of faculties (drives, energies, powers) within a given system. The elemental qualities of our body's system are part of a dynamic field and each elemental quality, as it presents itself, gives expression to the exact constellation of faculty that is present at the point at which the element is situated, a dynamic quality that permits the elemental qualities to become the conveyors of meaning; that makes temperaments out of the succession of elements.

Thus, we have introduced the traditional concepts of the soul and its place in space with the traditional components of space: structured (body, soul, spirit), oriented (six directions), sense of place (container/contained), positive space continuity (what flows through space creates shapes), time-form simultaneity (active as motion, passive as form), and rhythm in time (breath, pulse). Now let us turn to Avicenna. He begins *The Canon* with a definition of the science of medicine:

> Medicine (*tibb*) is the science by which we learn the various states of the human body in health and when not in health, and the means by which health is likely to be lost and, when lost, is likely to be restored back to health. In other words, it is the art whereby health is conserved and the art whereby it is restored after being lost.

Avicenna insists that the human body cannot be restored to health unless the causes of both health and disease are determined. In categorizing the causes, he uses Aristotle's system:

> Medicine deals with the states of health and disease in the human body. It is a truism of philosophy that a complete knowledge of a thing can only be obtained by elucidating its causes and antecedents, provided, of course, such causes exist. In medicine it is, therefore, necessary that causes of both health and disease should be determined.
>
> Sometimes these causes are obvious to the senses but at other times they may defy direct observation. In such circumstances, causes and antecedents have to be carefully inferred from the signs and symptoms of the disease. Hence, a description of the signs and symptoms of disease is also necessary for our purpose. It is a dictum of the exact sciences that knowledge of a thing is attained only through a knowledge of the causes and origins of the causes—assuming there to be causes and origins. Consequently our knowledge cannot be complete without an understanding both of symptoms and of the principles of being.

There are four causes—material, efficient, formal, and final. On the subject of health and disease, we have the following:

The Material Causes

The material (*maddi*) cause is the physical body which is the subject of health and disease. This may be immediate as the organs of body together with their vital energies and remote as the humours and remoter than these, the elements which are the basis both for structure and change (or dynamicity). Things which thus provide a basis (for health and disease) get so thoroughly altered and integrated that from an initial diversity there emerges a holistic unity with a specific structure (or the quantitative pattern of organization) and a specific type of temperament (the qualitative pattern).

The material cause, then is the physical body, as viewed from the traditional perspective. It consists of the organs, the breath, the humours and the elements. We begin with the elements as Avicenna does.

The Elements

The primary constituents of the human body in traditional medicine are called "the elements." They are the basic building blocks for the science of medicine.

The four elements—earth, air, fire, and water—are the simplest particles of all that is material. They are the simplest particles of our bodies. To each of them are joined two qualities. Earth is dry and cold; water, cold and moist; air, hot and moist; and fire is hot and dry. Earth is contrary to air and water to fire. Union is possible because water serves as a means between earth and air and air as a means between water and fire. The elements, like musical tones, possess an inclination not only to ascend and descend, but also to move in a circular direction. Each element is joined by one of its qualities to that which is below and by the other to that which is above it. Water to earth beneath by coldness and to air above by moisture; air to water beneath by moisture and to fire above by heat; fire to air beneath by heat and to earth toward which it declines by dryness; earth to water above by coldness and to fire which declines toward it by dryness. Two of the elemental qualities are active and two passive. Active are hot and cold. Passive are dry and wet. The resulting qualities, the ideal combination, is an equitable one.

Quality results from the opposing qualities of the elements, a mixture of hot, cold, wet and dry. Balance comes when the strength of primary qualities are equal to these qualities—an average of these qualities. In medicine, it does not depend upon exactly equal but "equitable," meaning that the quality and quantity of the elements are distributed in such a manner that the resulting pattern or equilibrium of the body as a whole or if its parts is the one most appropriate for that person.

When one quality predominates over the other, the body is not well suited to the needs of the soul. The proportion in which the elements are united with the body has an influence upon action. Slow and heavy moving signifies a predominance of cold and dryness (earth); fearfulness and sluggishness, of cold and wetness (water); cheerfulness, of heat and wetness (air); and sharp, angry violence, of heat and dryness (fire).

All physical forms consist of elemental qualities prefigured in the physical process. If something changes in the element, something must have changed in the physical process. The two stand to each other in the strict relationship of cause and effect.

As phenomena of the external world and, in traditional medicine, the inner world, consist of the elements and their qualities, as well. Different elemental qualities are always based on the different properties of the elements (higher, lower, lighter, heavier, colder, hotter, etc.). The distinguishing characteristic of the elements is that they differ like two colors, red and green, and like two shades of a single color, light and dark blue or like shapes rough and square. The property is a characteristic of such a nature that it both distinguishes different elements from one another and at the same time orders them in definite ways.

The dynamic quality of the elements is that they have direction. The elements point one to another—attract and are attracted—and are therefore directional forces. Elemental motion has its origin not in differences of properties but in differences of dynamic quality as conveyors of motion.

The Humours

The humours are the primary fluids of the body which move through inner space. These humours affect the function of the body and are themselves influenced by the states of motion and rest of the human being.

Food and drink are transformed into innate heat through the digestive process. The humours arise in the second stage of digestion in the liver. This process produces four humours which sustain and nourish the body and move through the channels or meridians: sanguineous (blood), serous (phlegm), bilious (choler, yellow bile) and atrabilious (melancholy, black bile) corresponding to air (hot and wet), water (cold and wet), fire (hot and dry) and earth (cold and dry). These are subject to variation in quantity and in degree of purity.

Illness results from either a quantitative or qualitative change of humour. In a "normal" state, the humours are assimilated by the organs and completely integrated into the tissues. In an "abnormal" state, due to improper digestion, the material is unsuitable for assimilation and therefore eliminated by the body. Surpluses may be eliminated by exercise, bathing, coition, purges and laxatives.

The sanguineous humour (blood), which is an equal temper, exceeds the others in proportion to quantity, is hot and moist, sweet and red. It imparts strength and color to the body and serves for the engendering of the drives. Located in the heart, it relates to Leo, Aries and Sagittarius in the Zodical constellations.

The serous humour or phlegm, next to blood in quantity, is watery, cold, moist and white. It moderates the strength, heat, and thickness of blood, nourishes the brain, and moistens and nourishes such part of the body as are concerned in motion. If blood fails, heat dissolves the serous humour into blood. Cancer, Pisces and Scorpio, as Zodiacal signs, relate to serous humour.

The bilious humour, least in quantity, is hot and dry, yellow or red and bitter. A part of it passes from the liver to the gallbladder and a part, flowing thence with other humours, moderates moisture and makes the blood subtle so that it may pass easily through straight ways. The bilious humour prevents the body from becoming heavy, sleepy and dull. It penetrates and opens passages and feeds members of the body in which the fiery element predominates. Zodiacal signs are Gemeni, Aquarius, and Libra.

The atrabilious humour is earthy and gross, thick, black and sour. A part of it passes to the spleen and a part remains with the blood. This humour feeds the bones, the spleen and other parts of the body which are gross or "melancholy" in nature. It tempers the two hot humours (sanguineous and bilious) and serves to stay and retain the floating spirits that arise from blood. The atrabilious humour thickens the blood and thus prevents it from flowing too freely through the veins and arteries. Within the Zodaic this humour is related to the three signs Tarus, Virgo, and Capricorn.

From the natural predominance of a humour in the human being spring definite characteristics of physique and conduct. Those dominated by the sanguinious humour are cheerful, courageous, kind and ingenious. Their blood, if subtle, makes the wit keen. As fatness increases, blood diminishes. The serous humour dominating is visible in people who are easily provoked, given to treachery and vehement in action; fierce in assailing but inconstant in sustaining the assault; inclined to envy, pride, prodigality and wrath. If the serous humour is corrupt, they are subject to evil passions and dreadful nightmares. Those with a predominance of bilious humour are generally slothful, given to bodily pleasures, sleepy, idle, dull of wit, heavy and slow. They love delicate food and drink. Those dominated by the atrabilious humour are hard to please, obstinate, suspicious, sorrowful and given to fearful thoughts.

The humours are exceedingly variable in quantity and quality. The sanguineous reigns from 3 am to 9 am; bilious from 9 am to 3 pm; serous from 3 pm to 9 pm and atrabilious from 9 pm to 3 am. The sanguineous humour increases in the spring. The heat of summer dissolves superfluities, wastes the humours and opens the pores. The breath escapes from the body with exhalations, moisture and vapors. The bilious humour is in ascendancy. Autumn breeds the serous humour.

Winter thickens the humours, constrains the sinews and sends natural heat inward. The atrabilious humour increases and makes people sluggish.

The active elemental qualities—cold and heat—form the humours. When heat is equable, the sanguineous humour forms; when heat is in excess, bilious humour forms; when in great excess so that oxidation occurs, atrabilious humour forms. When the cold is equable, serous humour forms; when cold is in excess so that congelation becomes dominant, atrabilious humour forms.

In addition to this, there are three souls within the human form:

> . . . namely, the vegetable, animal and rational, all of which descend from the world above and each of which possesses its own faculties. The more refined the mixture of the humours the greater the perfection and the more complete and perfect the possibility of receiving the soul. Moreover, in each man, health means the harmony of the humours and illness the disruption of the balance of the constitution. Of course the harmony is never perfect in any person, but relative to his own constitution, health means the re-establishment of the balance of the humours. Diagnosis for such disorders as fever are, in fact, based on searching for the way in which the balance of the humours has been upset. But for diseases which show overt signs, the most notable sign or signs are made use of it for diagnostic purposes and often the disease receives the name of the leading sign connected with it.[11]

Flowing in the space intermediate between the physical body and the force of life, is a placeless space, a space that, as a whole, has a direction and must have a center, the position toward which it is directed. Health or lack of it is is out from this center.

The Breath

The breath acts as the link between the body, soul and spirit. It is the breath which makes the perfect equilibrium of the elements possible.

God created the left side of the heart and made it hollow in order that it should serve both as a storehouse of the breath and as the seat of manufacture of the breath. He also created the breath to enable the drives of the "soul' to be conveyed into the corresponding members. In the first place the breath was to be the rallying-point for the faculties of the soul and in the second place it was to be an emanation into the various members and tissues of the body (whereby these could manifest the functions of those drives).

Now He produced the breath out of the finer particles of the humours and out of igneity and at the same time produced the tissues themselves (the visible body) out of the coarser and earthy particles of these humours. In other words, the breath is related to the attenuated particles as the body is related to the coarser particles of the same humours. Just as the humours are intermingled to produce a temperamental "form," whereby the members of the body are enabled to receive a physical appearance, impossible were they separate, so the attenuated portions of the humours, being intermingled into a temperamental form, enable the breath to receive the powers of the soul—impossible were the humours separate.

The beginning of the breath is as a divine emanation from potentiality to actuality proceeding without intermission or stint until the form (preparation, state) is completed and perfected. Each member, though derived from the self-same substance of the humours, nevertheless has its own particular temperament—for the proportional qualities of the (denser portions of the) humours and the form of their commixture are peculiar to each member. Similarly, although derived from the same attenuated portions of the humours, nevertheless each of the three breaths (natural, animal and vital) has its own particular temperament, because the proportional quantities of the more attenuated portions of the humours and the manner of their commixture are peculiar to each breath.

Although the body consists of several organs, there is one from which they all originally arose. As to what this organ actually was, there are various opinions. The fact remains that one organ necessarily came to light before other organs could arise out of it. Exactly the same is true in the case of the breaths. There is one single breath which accounts for the origin of the others. This breath, according to the most important philosophers, arises in the heart, passes thence into the principal centers of the body, lingering in them long enough to enable them to impart to it their respective temperamental properties. Lingering in the cerebrum it receives a temperament whereby it is capable of receiving the drives of sensation and movement; in the liver, it receives the drive of nutrition and growth (vegetative drives); in the generative glands it acquires a temperament which prepares it for receiving the drive of generation (reproduction).

The breath is similar to the spirit and is of three kinds:

(1) The vital spirit, hot and dry, has its center in the left ventricle of the heart, preserves life, causes the body to grow, move and reproduce, and travels through the arteries. (2) The psychic spirit, cold and wet, has its center in the brain, causes sensation and movement and moves through the nerves and is the source of movement and reason. (3) The natural spirit, hot and wet, has its center in the liver, is concerned with the reception of food, growth and reproduction and travels through the veins.[12]

Traditional medicine is first concerned with the rhythmic continuity of the breath itself and then the synthesis of breath as "time in motion" or "active space" and organs or members as "passive possibilities of space" of matter and form. Harmonic order brings together those two concepts of breath and organs which appear to be opposite but which inwardly contain one another and are therefore complements. The synthesis is achieved because the breath occupies a continuous space defined by passageways, meridians, channels which move through the shapes of organs, bones, muscles. Movement coalesces breath and organs into a unity.

The Organs

The humours in turn act as the constituent elements for the members or organs of the body which "are derived primarily from the commingling of the humours, just as the humours are derived primarily from the commingling of the aliments and the aliments are primarily composed of commingled elements. The organs are divided into simple ones having homogeneous parts such as flesh, bones, and nerves, and compound organs such as the hands and face. The organs are the instruments by which the passions and actions of the mind are achieved and act as its servants.

The primary elemental quality of an organ is based on its nutrient while its secondary quality is determined by what it excretes.

Hot organs consist of the vital force and heart, blood, liver, flesh, muscle, spleen, kidneys, breasts, testicles, muscular coats of arteries, veins, skin of palm (which is evenly balanced).

Cold organs consist of phlegm, hair, bones, cartilage, ligaments, serous membranes, nerves, spinal cord, brain, solid and liquid fats and skin.

Moist organs consist of phlegm, blood, sold and liquid fats, brain, spinal cord, breast, testicles, lungs, liver, spleen, kidneys, muscles, and skin.

Dry organs consist of hair, bones, cartilage, ligaments, tendons, membranes, arteries, veins, motor nerves, heart, sensory nerves, skin.

The Efficient Causes

> The efficient (*failiya*) causes are capable of either preventing or inducing change in the human body. They may be external to the person or internal. External causes are: age, sex, occupation, residence, and climate and other agents which effect the human body by contact whether contrary to nature or not. Internal causes are sleep and wakefulness, evacuation of secretions and excretions, the changes at different periods of life in occupation, habits and customs, ethnic group and nationality.

The efficient causes are clear and vary with each individual. Whereas the elements, humours, breath and organs as the material cause are all from nature, the efficient causes develop out of the nurturing process.

The Formal Causes

> The formal (*suriyah*) causes are three: temperaments (*mizajat*) (or the pattern of constitution as a whole) and the faculties or drives (*qawa*) which emerge from it and the structure (the quantitative patterns).

Temperament

Temperament arises from the elements and humours and it determines the way in which the soul functions. Each animal and each organ of the body has a temperament of its own.

> The Almighty Creator has bestowed upon every animal and every one of its organs the most appropriate and the best adapted temperament for its various functions and passive states.
>
> Since the verification of this truth is a matter for philosophers and not physicians, we may accept that the human being has been bestowed a most befitting temperament and most appropriate faculty or drives for the various active and passive states in the body. Similarly, every organ and member is endowed with the proper temperament appropriate to its own functional requirement. Some He has made more hot, others more cold, others more dry and others more moist.

The temperament is "equable" when the contrary qualities are in perfect equilibrium, and out of harmony or "inequable" when the temperament tends toward a particular quality. Therapeutics, then, are based on the allopathic principle of contraries. That is, "cold" diseases can be cured by "hot" remedies and vice versa.

Avicenna then explains this method further:

> It is worth remembering that when a medicine is referred to as being evenly balanced, it does not mean that its temperament is the same as of a human being, or that it is even similar to it, for it would then be like a human being. It merely means that such a medicine, after being acted upon by the innate heat [metabolized] fails to produce any material change in the normal state of the body, and that its pharmacological actions remain within the limits of normal human temperament. In other words, when this medicine is given to a normal person, it does not produce any appreciable change or imbalance in the body. When it is said that a drug is hot or cold, it does not mean that the physical quality of the drug is particularly hot or cold or that it is colder or hotter than the human body. If this were so there would follow the unwarranted inference mentioned above that an evenly constituted medicine is the one which has exactly the same temperament as the human body. It means just that such a medicine produces a greater amount of heat or cold than what was originally present in the body. A drug which, for example, is cold for the human being may be hot for the scorpion, or the medicine which is hot for the human being may be cold for the serpent. In fact it may also mean that the same medicine may be less hot for one person than for another. This is the reason why physicians are advised to change their medicine when it fails to produce the desired result.

The growth and decay of the human body is dependent upon the human temperament. Growth depends upon the heat contained in the sperm which is gradually used up. Meanwhile, the moisture lessens in quantity and quality, thus preserving the innate heat at a constant level up to the old age. Ultimately, however, the moisture of the body comes to an end, and the innate heat i.e. extinguished, thus causing the death to which everyone is destined and which depends upon the original temperament of the human body.

The correspondences between the various orders of reality and the temperament have been summed up in the following:

> The uniqueness of the temperament of each individual indicates that each microcosm is a world of its own, not identical with any other microcosm. Yet, the repetition of the same basic humours in each constitution bears out the fact that each microcosm presents a morphological resemblance to other microcosms. Moreover, there is an analogy between the human body and the cosmic order, as shown by the correspondence between the humours and elements. There is in the Hermetico-alchemical natural philosophy, which was always closely tied

to medicine in Islam, a basic doctrine of the correspondence between all the various orders of reality: the intelligible hierarchy, the heavenly bodies, the order of numbers, the parts of the body, the letters of the alphabet which are the "elements" of the Sacred Book, etc. The seven cervical and the twelve dorsal vertebrae correspond to the seven planets and the twelve signs of the Zodiac, as well as to the days of the week and the months of the year; and the total number of discs of the vertebrae, which they consider to be twenty-eight, to the letters of the Arabic alphabet and the stations of the moon. There is, therefore, both numerical and astrological symbolism connected with medicine, although the closeness of the relation has not been the same during all periods of Islamic history, nor among all the medical authorities. But the correspondence and "sympathy" (in the original sense of the word "sympathia") between various orders of cosmic reality form the philosophical background of Islamic medicine.[13]

The Faculties or Drives

The body also possesses faculties which originate the functions of various organs. The major faculties are (1) the vital (*hayawaniyah*), responsible for preserving the integrity of the breath, sensation, and movement of the heart; (2) the natural (*tabiiyah*) governing the nutritive powers of the liver and the reproductive powers of the generating organs; and (3) the animal (*nafsaniyah*) controlling the brain and the rational faculty.

The powers of the various members are due to the vital faculty[14] which provides the body with its inner force. The vital faculty is that which appears in the breath at the very moment at which the breath develops out of the rarefied particles of the humours.

Between the human body as a whole and the individual points as its parts there is a relationship—the whole being given with and active in the part and the part being aware that it is part and directly announcing its relation to the whole. Whenever we encounter a phenomenon showing this relationship between whole and parts we may assume, that a force, an ordered action of forces, is the basis. This is the role of the faculties which we can only know through their effects. They work through the physical body without ever touching it.

The Final Causes

The final (*tamamia*) causes are the actions or functions. They can be understood only from a knowledge of both the faculties or drives (*qawa*) and the vital energies (breaths, *arwah*) that are ultimately responsible for them. These will be described presently.

IV. Conclusion

The power of traditional Islamic medicine is in realizing that space leads and forms shapes; shapes then interact with space and space with the breath/inner light with which every human being has been endowed. What he or she does with that determines the extent of their completion and perfection.

O. Cameron Gruner's Remarks

During the past fifty years,[1] the popular imagination has been stirred by a succession of important discoveries in the domain of medicine and surgery. The triumphs of the latter field have been spectacular to a degree. Those of medicine have been much less conspicuous, chiefly because the mind must inquire into them before it can properly appreciate them. How much does not humanity owe to the steadily continued researches in bacteriology, and the painstaking observations which have revealed the life-cycles of many of the parasites to which tropical and other diseases are due and to the whole procedure of immuno-therapy, the just pride of scientific as distinct from clinical medicine, and the outcome of all these researches?

As compared with all this, the speculative subtleties of former times appear both futile and unworthy of resuscitation. But the ancient system was not as valueless as is so generally supposed. Taking as an adequate criterion the first book of *The Canon of Medicine* of Avicenna, which is here presented [almost in its entirety], and is fairly representative of the whole work, we find in its pages references to many departments of human knowledge—(though it might be objected that all these departments of knowledge are now separate sciences, each requiring its own professorial staff, its own literature, and journals and that they are not mentioned under the special names with which we are familiar, their existence in those days cannot be denied) cosmology, anatomy, physiology, and psychology; the: various branches of clinical medicine-etiology, semiology, diagnosis, and prognosis; the departments of therapeutics-hygiene, dietetics, balneology, and climatology, in addition to materia medica, pharmacology, and pharmacy. Moreover, the reader is presumed to be conversant with logic, criteriology, and metaphysics.

The presence of obvious literal errors in the work must not lead us to commit the more serious mistake of overlooking the fact that it is entirely built up upon a sound philosophy of human nature, which is as vitally important today, though largely ignored in former times. The traditional medicine was concerned essentially with the given patient now before us; whereas now it is simply the science of diseases which it is our duty to diagnose accurately, prevent if possible, and treat on lines capable of wholesale application. To Avicenna, the determination of the constitution of the patient was of the very first importance, because on it depended the character, course, and duration of his illness, and upon that again depended the choice of remedies.

After all, from the patient's point of view, the real object of consulting a medical man is to be restored to a state of well-being. It is little comfort to be virtually told that 85-90 percent of cases of his complaint are cured by the treatment adopted in his case, only to find that he proves to be one of the remaining 10-15 percent for whom there is little or nothing to be done. True, his sighs are drowned in the shouts of the fortunate, and fail to reach the clinical laboratory, surgical wards, consulting room or research councils.

If, in the interests of these few, chance leads us to the pages of this traditional work, it would seem that suggestions occur in it which enable us to understand their plight, and thereby help them to understand it also. Even if the enemy is not put out of action, his enmity is less evident when he is understood.

It has been the aim of this treatise to elaborate Avicenna's central theme by references to the various philosophies extant in his time—Sufi, Vedantic, Buddhist, Chinese; to Persian writings subsequent to his time (Rumi, Sadi, Shabistari, etc.); and to views presented by various modern philosophies, including western theosophy.

But these various directions of thoughts are not drawn upon in order to elaborate a composite system after the fashion of theosophical eclecticism. On the contrary, readers accustomed to various modes of thought are invited across a bridge leading from their various starting-points, across the chasm of modernism, until they reach the concise teaching of Thomistic philosophy, wherein all other aspects of the one truth receive their proportionate places. The inclusion of ideas from writers whose ideas appear to be altogether of the by-ways may torment a few, but may also help a few to see the: greater thing, and thereafter be content to stay upon the broad highway to which the several paths have converged.

Science has been removed from its usual role of master, and has been pressed into service, and that service is to illuminate the subject of human nature. To quote a recent paper,[2] "Under the great swelling flood that represents the growing complexity of modern medicine, let us not allow ourselves hold fast to that great life-saving conception of the essential unity of the human body. Let us oppose fearlessly those currents of medical thought that tend to isolate—arbitrarily and to the detriment of true knowledge—the various segments of this one great subject. Let us welcome all methods, all discoveries, that help the one man in charge of the one patient to broaden the base of his attack, to widen the sweep of his beneficent vision." These words were possibly expressed with a different object, but apply well to the theme of this treatise.

The old teaching about "constitution" should undergo a mutual inter-growth with the knowledge of modern science, pervaded throughout with the fundamental teaching of Thomistic philosophy, when there would emerge the beginnings of a possible system of modern scholastic medicine—thoroughly logical, plain, free of mystery, free of materialism, but not ignoring the so-called "occult" and metaphysical; with the knowledge of the nature of the constitution of the individual patient as its central and dominant theme. Were the whole medical training along such lines, the student would be able to approach his clinical instruction thoroughly aware that the individuality of the patient comes first, and that the ailment from which he suffers is but part and parcel of one single story, and not merely an accidental superposition. But the student would constantly need guidance to ensure his over-riding the disregard or ignorance, if not actual rejection, of scholastic principles which characterizes the concrete modern teaching of pathology in its various departments.

The following brief survey of the most important teachings of *The Canon.*

Teachings of The Canon

The General Notion of the Nature of a Human Being

The following three propositions belong to it: (1) the human being (MF)[3] is composed of matter and a principle of life, the two together making him "he" or "she," he or she is "a single substance endowed with a natural tendency to realize and maintain the conditions of its organization." (2) This principle of life comprises three main groups of potential and actual activities—the vegetative, the sensitive and the rational. This multi-potentiality of the principle of life is represented in the expression "bundle of life." (3) The organs of the body are the material manifestations (the actualities) of the several potentialities The vegetative organs belong to the "vegetative soul," the sense-organs and appurtenances belong to the "sensitive soul." The intelligence and will belong to the "rational soul," which has not literal organs but acts through the instrumentation of the organs of the vegetative and sensitive systems. All these components belong intimately together apart from macroscopic or microscopic boundaries it.

These propositions are further defined by the following negative statements: (1) the human being is not a collection of molecules and forces; he manifests chemical, electric, and other phenomena, which are not causes, but effects. (2) The organs are not distinct from the powers they exhibit. (3) The brain is not the producer of thought.

The remarkable action which the human being achieves by his complicated mechanical contrivances are distinct from himself, whereas in the human being the mechanism and the manipulator are the self same. Even when there is as grave mechanical interference with organs as occurs in hemiplegia, or in the cortical lesions of insanity, the rational soul remains untouched, though no longer able to communicate its activities to the outer world. To quote from St. Thomas, "The intellect, being a power that does not make use of a corporeal organ, would in no way be hindered in its act through the lesion of a corporeal organ, if for its act there were not required the act of some power that does make used of a corporeal organ."[4]

Thought is produced by the activity of the rational souls; the changes in the brain—whether chemical, cytological, or otherwise—are not causes, but the visible effects of the activity. (4) There is no bridge over the gulf between rational life and the-vegetative sensitive life; the distinctions are radical. (5) The life-principle is not subject to the laws of inheritance, those which govern matter; it is not divisible into organs, or parts, or elements. As soon as it ceases to operate, it is left behind the material body, which though apparently the same is actually quite different from the animate person recently before me.

The Notion of the Constitution of Any Given Individual When in Health

This notion should be made as tangible as possible.[5] The constitution may be expressed in terms of a number of formula to be taken together—a series of "notes," some of which are constants, and others variables. In this formula, the qualities are represented by the initials of their corresponding names; the quantities are represented by index numbers from 1 to 5, to stand for slight, moderate, normal, marked, and very marked, and very marked respectively.

The Constants

I. *The Body:* (1) general physique [good, poor, robust, spare, strong, delicate]; (2) dominant "element" [example: $E^2W^2F^5A^3$] for earth, water, fire and air; (3) dominant "humour," shown in the humoural formula [example: $S^3L^1B^5A^8$] for sanguineous, serous (lymphatic), bilious, and atrabilious]. This formula is really descriptive of the "temperament," but the latter word bears a different meaning in modern popular usage. (4) The absolute or relative strength or weakness (functional capacity) of the several organs; hypo, hyper-function. [example: $V^4T^4M^20^3N^1lG^3$, for vegetative (i.e. alimentary), thoracic (i.e. respiratory and circulatory), muscular (including skeletal), osseous (including genito-urinary), nervous (including sympathetic system) and glandular (including haemopoietic, endocrine, and hepatic) types. (5) The emotional make-up, or formula [example: $G^3L^2T^1I^5$ (gaudium, laetitia, timor, ira),[6] from which the dominant passion and its modifiers are noted. The modern use of the word "temperament" belongs here.

The difference in capacity is partly explained by considering the time-factor,[7] and partly as a fundamental difference.[8] All the material brought to an organ, whether nutritive, or excretory, is not at once taken up in its entirety; only a certain proportion is removed and the remainder passes on, so that the blood has its composition at a certain level. The modern threshold values recognize this fact. The time-factor is of very great importance.

II. *The Mind:* here comes the description of the disposition, the type of mind, or mental make-up.[9] Mental capacity may be expressed in terms of the relative or absolute strength or weakness of the various faculties, enumerated under "talents" (which are simply developments of particular faculties above the average).[10]

> "The better the disposition of a body, the better the soul allotted to it which clearly appears in things of different species: and the reason thereof is that act and form are received into matter according to matter's capacity thus because some men have bodies of better disposition, their souls have a greater power of understanding . . . . This occurs in regard to the lower powers of which the intellect has need in its operation, because those in whom the imaginative, cogitative and memorative powers are of better disposition, are better disposed to understand."[11]

The mental attitude towards things, which emerges from the character, is also to be noted, for sometimes this may explain the cause of the illness (i.e., wanton exposure to infections in spite of warnings), and will show whether the patient is suppressing relevant facts, will respond to treatment, or is secretly concerned with some fear or doubt which is the real object of his visit to the doctor. Moreover, knowledge of this aspect of character will safeguard the physician himself, either by making him aware of the patient's possible cynical opinion about a profession he is unfortunately obliged to deal with, or, more important, by enabling him to avoid offering advice which is palpably foolish to an intelligent patient.

The Variables

The degree of vitality: this is also spoken of as the strength of innate heat in the text;[12] (2) deviations from the functional capacities normal to the individual; (3) the nature or degree of "resistance." In terms of *The Canon*, this would be expressed in the "humoural formula," and in terms of "obstructions" of various kinds. These account for the "soil" which renders declared disease: (a) possible; or (b) amenable to alteration by artificial means.[13]

Foreign though such data are to modern clinical work, they are often actually employed in ordinary conversation, as when one describes a person as sanguine, or bilious, or phlegmatic, or as of saturnine temperament. Some adjective descriptive of the emotional make-up is not infrequent in case reports degrees of vitality are spoken of seriously by the laity, diplomatically by the practitioner.

In so far as they provide a simple means of codifying tentative knowledge upon complex and elusive individual characteristics which it is our duty to notice, the data are all worth consideration.

The Notion of the Nature of the State of Disease

The vegetative processes associated with digestion and absorption of food may be first briefly referred to. The picture of the whole nutritive cycle is comprehended in the idea of the "liver."[14] We trace the food constituents through the columnar cells of the intestinal mucosa, across the areolar tissue into the vascular roots of the portal and lacteal system; then into the liver unit itself (comprising phagocytic secretary cells, fundal cells, cubical excretory cells, and the hepatic arterioles and lymphatic clefts related to the sinusoids); then into the general blood-stream, and finally out of the body through various organs, including the goblet cells of the intestinal mucosa, the bile-ducts, the pancreas, etc. The extra-hepatic portion of the cycle is nearly co-terminous with the rest of the body.

To complete this picture we first remember the relation between the quality of food and the quality of chyme; then we consider how the ultimate components of the food travel (N-compounds, glucose, fat, phosphorus, sulphur, iron, and the like)—during rest, exercise, sleep, etc. and according to the character of the diet as a whole, the fluids taken, and the state of the bowels, etc. We may realize that they are manifested in the blood in the form of alkaline tide, viscosity, fibrin-content, and the various morphological changes revealed by blood-examination. We picture also the innumerable chemical interchanges and physical transformations in various parts of the cycle; the formation of waste-substances, and the factors on which the whole of the processes depend. [15] In brief, then our picture of the body is that of a complex of tubes and channels —potential as well as actual—which vary in size from the obvious alimentary-canal, air-passages, and great blood vessels, down to the finest ramifications of the latter, the cavernous tissues—both macroscopic and microscopic—the serous cavities, and the intracellular channels. All these form one continuous labyrinthine system, through which we may trace the ingested food materials, the metabolic, secretory and excretory products. As long as these channels are patent throughout, and As long as these various subs stances (including the "breath of life") can flow freely through them, and the vital energy has a free play outward, so long is the body in a state of health.

But as soon as there is a continued interference with the freedom of movement, even though it be merely an ebb and flow that is affected, in any part of the canalicular system, then a state of disease arises, culminating in histological anatomical changes. Hence, when we observe a case of illness, we may be sure there is some "obstruction" in some channels in some part of the body—not necessarily in that where the symptoms occur (i.e., the nasal discharge of "cold in the head," the bronchial expectoration in bronchitis, the serous effusion into the pleura, the respiratory phenomena in an attack of asthma, are manifestations in the respiratory system of obstructions elsewhere).

The next addition to the picture of the sick person's state is furnished by the causes of the obstruction. Avicenna considered these under two groups, the "'material" (i.e. those in which "matter" is concerned) or "humoural diseases" and the non-material. To the latter group would belong cases of gross obstruction, such as by compression from without, or such as by obstruction with calculi and those in which there is a functional disorder—hypo-function, hyper-function, dysfunction. For instance, in renal disease, the loss of functional capacity may render the-normal ebb and flow of substances disorderly.[16]

The group of humoural diseases is predominant in Avicenna's pathology, and if we bear in mind what the "humours" really are, this position becomes quite reasonable. Perverted metabolism is associated with changes of physical state in the fluids of the body. Limpid fluids may become viscid, viscous substances may become mobile or "tenuous." In the ancient work, these chemical changes were thought of, not in "equations," but under interchanges between the imponderable elements, as being subject to the laws of *uruj, nasul, jalal, jamal, qada, qadr*,[17] the rhythm, phases and rate of movement of the "breath" and the fluctuations of degrees of innate heat. Concrete examples are such as: precipitation of urates in tissues, altered reaction of tissue juices in rheumatoid arthritis, cardio-renal disease, tuberculosis; variations of content of Ca, Na, Mg, etc., in the tissue-water, so that the flow from tissue to blood and vice versa is impeded.[18]

The Canon often insists on the presence of "superfluities" as a cause of "obstructions" of the canalicular system not only in the tangible four humours, but also in regard to the "breath."[19] In the latter case, the substance of the breath (i.e. water-vapor) ceases to be "bright," and "clear," and its odor becomes offensive, and its freedom of flow is impaired .

Finally, adding from modern knowledge, there are the changes in the fluids of the body produced by bacterial or putrefactive breakdown—whether this begins in intestinal stasis or arises in the course of specific bacterial infections. There are then obstructions not only in the old sense, but in the form of the successive histological lesions consequent—vascular, nutritional, and inflammatory. Materials are deposited more or less permanently (irreversible reactions), as i.e., solid odema, collagenous tissue, scar formation, fibrosis, and hyalo-fibrosis, adipose tissue, hyperplastic formations. Loss of anatomical patency is super added to loss of functional perviousness.

Clearly, whereas we give first place to the bacterial invasion, Avicenna gave it to the habits of life. He was deeply impressed by the obvious fact that the quality of food determines the kind of chyme, and that the kind of chyme determines the quality of the freedom of flow through the diffuse canalicular system of the body. As they accumulate in the stagnating tissue-juices they come to exercise a noxious action; they come to be beyond the capacity of the third and fourth digestions (tissue-digestion), and with their stagnation, the ever-circulating bacteria (taken up with the food) also settle and multiply and wandering-cell infiltrations gather together. The beginnings of disease are laid down. The functional disturbance has been succeeded by anatomical lesions.[20]

Finally, Avicenna enlarges his view of humoural disease by noting the influence of many extracorporeal factors[21] as well as the period of life, not to mention "the decree of God."[22] Thus, one and the same kind of food taken at the "warm" period of life in the "warm" season may contribute more to the formation of a given humour than at another.

If we knew the patient's formula, and how the climactic and other conditions are likely to affect it, and whether they are compatible or not with susceptibility to the agents at work, our composite picture of the patient's state would be of great value, and illnesses often inexplicable would lose their mystery. How much more efficient might not the treatment be, if the remedial measures in contemplation were selected to harmonize with them?

No doubt only a fanatic would note the barometer, thermometer, humidity, hours of sunshine, wind-direction and velocity, the character of previous seasons, the clues afforded by then migration so insects, rodents, and birds, the presence or prevalence of certain parasites in a district, and the many other points noted in Part Three[23] before prescribing the regimen for the patient. But it would seem that some Eastern physicians of bygone times conscientiously strove to learn from such factors.

The Guides to the Diagnosis of the State of the Patient

The patient before us is as a manuscript written in some highly complex language which it is our business to decipher. The alphabet is furnished by the several colors, the simple observations of size, shape, consistency, contour, texture, and the like. The vocabulary consists of the external features both in repose and animation, and of the physical signs as taught to-day. The grammar lies in the "general guides" (sphygmology, urinoscopy, examination of feces and blood). The language is to be translated into: states of natural (vegetative), sensitive, and emotional instinctive drives, functional capacities, plethora, obstructions, solutions of continuity, etc. that is, the state of the whole composite, in all aspects. This task can only be accomplished imperfectly at the best, even by the most skilled and most learned. Our silent teachers, or guides, the "indications" always enable us to ascertain something, and we must perforce be content with that on the present occasion and be determined to use this experience as the guide to better success on the next.

One of the guides suggested in *The Canon* lies in one's own state of health. Properly to interpret what we observe, we must ourselves have no disharmony of functions arising from errors of diet, no deposit in the urine, no weight in the bowels, no obstructions in our own brain, no mental fatigue, no emotional pre-occupation, no rigid notions regarding etiology or prognosis; there must be clear channels for the breath, and the breath must be under the control of the will. It must be kept pure by recollection, by devotion, and observance of prayer. The reason for this is that under such conditions, long persevered, we are enabled to receive an "impression" from the patient. We become aware of his atmosphere, aura, or personality in the form of an idea of his degree and kind of vitality. But unless this impression is registered rapidly, namely at the first approach of the patient, it will be confused and illegible by reason of the mutual inter-impression of one's own vitality with his. In another idiom, we observe "with the eye of a Taoist." In our own idiom, we make use of sound reasoning power, common sense, and a certain kind of "intuition," or "clinical sense."

The guides furnished by general observation of the patient are, in brief: (1) external features in repose: (a) colors of face, hair, skin, eye (sclerae, iris); (b) odors and savors; (c) form of the body: (i) as a whole; (ii) in detail. The features, the hands, the limbs; the relative proportions (length, breadth, and thickness) of nose, cheeks, upper lip, lower lip, chin, mouth, ears, orbit, eyebrows, forehead, etc.; the character of the neck, shoulders, etc. (2) Features when animated: (a) expression, gaze, look, facial gestures (vivacity, sleepiness, languidness); (b) deportment or attitude,[24] gestures, carriage, specific acts or mannerisms, definitely morbid movements or defective movements. (c) voice: tone of voice, manner of speech (clear, loud, or the opposite); clues to the physical and mental type, and the degree of energy and vitality.

Space does not allow of any attempt to furnish precise details of the external signs of functional capacity of internal organs. The principle is exemplified thus: the lower part of the nose is part of the respiratory system, and shares in the degree of development of the whole system; therefore wide nostrils with well-formed aloe go with good development of the whole respiratory function, whereas narrow delicate nostrils and small alae refer the observer to some other system as well-developed. Large mouth, thick lips, large masseters, and generally well-developed lower part of the face go with good development of the digestive tract throughout. Moreover, development or capacity above the average in one system denotes relative weakness and functional deficiency in another system. The subject is extensive.[25]

Our general guides differs noticeably, from that revealed in *The Canon*. To follow Avicenna, (1) when one places the hand on the pulse, one absorbs oneself in it, without the distraction of a watch, until one has found out how it runs minute after minute. Even if it misses, without an intermission of the heart, because the patient gives a twitch of the finger or begins to talk, one learns even from that. The study of the circulation is more than the study of the heart's action. (2) When one examines the urine, even with all the apparatus of modern chemistry, we must remember that it is first and foremost the guide to the state of digestion—especially its "second stage" (that in the liver) as well as in the "third" stage (that in the small vessels). We are misled by the search for albuminuria and glycosuria, for many would make these abnormalities into diseases. Thus, the number of persons in whom albuminuria is not evidence of renal disease far outnumber those in which it is; the presence of such a substance in the urine should lead to the questions: is some substance not being dealt with? If so, why? Can only the kidney handle it? To follow a useful rule, the real trouble is remote. It may lie in the brain, in the emotional state (cf. Graves' disease, i.e., pentosuria, cystinuria, alkaptonuria also break the current ideas about urinalysis.[26] (3) As regards the guide furnished by the feces matter, again, our knowledge is much greater than was Avicenna's and we do not apply it in his terms. We are apt to lose ourselves in fat analyses, nitrogen estimations, occult blood tests, B. coli classifications. Negative results in each case are taken to mean nothing of note, regardless of the continual secretory and excretory changes proceeding in the intestinal mucosa, and the vitality of nerve-ganglia, etc. Essential and definite derangements may occur without conspicuous deviations from the restricted standards usually laid down.

The guide furnished by an examination of the brood may be spoken of as the most notable modern addition to Avicenna's three general guides. The data obtained from it—physical, physicochemical, cytological, serological—are very numerous, but are lost more often than not by restriction to the diagnosis of the various "blood-diseases." When properly applied, all the data obtained from the blood inform us of the functional state of all the organs and of the existence of the main groups of pathological state.[27]

Treatment

"The healing art, as it is described in books, is far inferior to the practical experience of a skillful and thoughtful physician." (Rhazes).

"Many are healed by the action of nature without the art of medicine."[28] "Man teaches by outward ministration, but God by inward operation: even so the physician is said to minister, to nature when he heals."[29]

Application of the principles of *The Canon* to modern practice would seem superfluous. The common ailments, especially those of minor surgery, are nowadays treated in stereotyped fashion, which appears to be beyond improvement. It is not with such cases that reference to *The Canon* is suggested. It is the general principle which may be reviewed in the mind, and lines of treatment such as were once in vogue may be quite usefully applicable in a few cases which do not well respond to modern methods. Moreover, the conscience of even the most careful may not be altogether clear in regard to the immemorial rule: "*tutto, cito, et jucunde*."

The subject may be briefly considered under two headings: plan of treatment; methods of treatment.

The Plan of Treatment

The choice of a plan of treatment depends on the view which is taken as to the cause of the illness. It is no new or modern thing to say "treat the cause." The distinction between new and old is in regard to the idea of the nature of the cause. In these days nearly every illness is ultimately due to an infection or intoxication, and the aim of treatment is to destroy the one and render the other innocuous. To Avicenna, illness was primarily an abnormal state of condition, to which many factors contributed. The scheme of treatment must, therefore, envisage them all. To facilitate this, the practitioner of those days would advisedly mentally review the whole of the second part.[30]

Indeed, if we scrutinize the subject more closely, it will appear that Avicenna's plan is after all very proper. For, even if we could attack the microbic cause specifically, there would still remain the lesions which it has produced, and the lowering of the vitality (=interferences with the flow of vital currents, in Paracelsus' idiom)[31] A condition remains to be combated; the condition is uppermost as far as the patient is concerned. Even in those relatively few cases in which the disease is bound up-with a particular organ, so that the name of the disease is according (i.e., gastric ulcer, cerebral hemorrhage), it is the condition we have to face. The cause, even when known, has done its work, and gone.

It is true that many other interpretations of disease and corresponding plans of treatment are put forward in various quarters from time to time, especially by the intellectually anarchistic. This occurrence is partly the outcome of the arbitrary attitudes towards patient and friends sometimes exhibited by some of the representatives of academic medicine and would be best met by frank and courteous enquiry into lay opinions. Not everyone subscribes to the restrictions of medical ethics, and the patient is too often treated as if illness ipso facto at once deprives him of ordinary intelligence. After all, he seeks medical help for a distinct object, and remuneration for the services is presumed, so that he is entitled to go elsewhere, at his own choice, if unfortunately in his particular case the plan and method of treatment proves unsuccessful. But this view is not subscribed to by those who assume that the whole of the knowledge needed for every case is comprehended within the orthodox teaching of the day, and that every individual possesses.

The Methods of Treatment

Even the methods of treatment set forth in The Canon are still resorted to at times. No doubt, we would do well to follow them more frequently. Thus, systematic purgation is often called for, but not carried out as radically as of old. Cupping is still of value for such conditions as lumbar myositis, acute hemorrhagic nephritis, and those diseases amenable to autohaemolysins. Venesection is sometimes effectively applied for cases of high blood-pressure, threatened apoplexy; it is incidentally used in the course of obtaining blood-tests.

Drug Treatment

The steady decline of drug treatment in modern medical practice is evidenced in several directions: (1) the steady removal, in successive editions of the *British Pharmacopceia* of herbal remedies which are supposed to have no action because laboratory animals appear to be unaffected by them; (2) the infrequency with which medicines are ordered for hospital patients; (3) the penalization of panel practitioners for "over-prescribing"; (4) the desire on the part of many lay persons to banish "drugs" as being "unnatural."

Inconsistencies are frequent. There is the strange perversity which (through legislation) denies facilities for the use of the few drugs whose potency is quite unquestionable. There is the subterfuge of resorting to placebos (which often cost no more than the bottle containing them). Those among the lay who decry drugs are pleased to employ herbal remedies. Where there is a popular demand for the latest remedies, this is met by a never-ending stream of new synthetic and other preparations, and costly manufactured products, which also the medical world submits to. Truly the mind ever seeks in the relatively inaccessible, and the expensive, that which lies all the time, and without price, at our feet. It describes as progress that which better knowledge would render superfluous.

The truth is that we know far too little about the herbal remedies of *The Canon*. To begin with we forget that they cannot be efficient without careful attention to the conditions of their cultivation (soil, climate, season, etc.), the times proper for their collections, the details of their preservations and the laws governing the formation and circulation of the active principles during the life-cycles of the various plants. We do not individually know how to identify adulterations, whether accidental or deliberate. We leave to wholesale manufacture that which was once properly undertaken individually since personal artistic skill may be the real condition for pharmacological efficiency. We adopt the short cut of standardization of drugs as the remedy for the loss of potency inevitable after neglect of such various factors. But even if the purity and potency of remedies be granted, by recourse to the best sources they must be employed with deliberate care.

As Avicenna shows in the second book of *The Canon*, there must be a knowledge of the constitution or individuality of the plants which yield the drug; harmony with the constitution of the patient must be aimed at. Out of a number of drugs of like action, some will accord better with one person as constitution than with another's. One remedy may soothe and ease without its specific action being at all diminished whereas another performs its work harshly and unpleasantly; another may be overpowered by the personal factor. The scope of the subject is great and its study with intent to serious practical application, should not require an apologia.

Such considerations as these open the door of romance. The discovery that all nature is a living whole, always at work, earnestly, steadily, continuously developing an fidea, would arouse a new and intensely absorbing interest—that of watching the unseen worker, though His hands are not to be discerned, that which He does is ever proceeding before us as a continual motion-picture, and we may become aware not only of the merely superficial fact of the movements, but also of the purpose unfolding.

Watching the medicinal trees and shrubs and herbs in this way, and seeing their properties by their forms, and colors and odors, and their changes in character with the changes of the seasons, and alternations of drought and plenty (variations of rate of growth, of activity of flowering and fruiting), how great is the wonder of the work of nature! We note how substances are being elaborated into plants which we, wanting their help, know how to take at the crucial moment—now we must draw the resin; now we must take these flowering tops, and so on. But we are not the only watchers. The bees have been waiting, the birds, the slugs, the ants, the herbivora all these and many others wait to draw from such supplies that which is applicable to their several requirements. Nature itself also waits for all these things to be collected from its treasury. Everything has been worked out; the interactions are arranged for they all belong to the purpose of the Designer; and He Himself is waiting for that over which He incessantly broods, with entire and complete intention. He too waits to draw out of Creation that which was His object in making it.

No doubt it is true that few of the ancient physicians entered fully into this inner life of the world of which they formed a part. Few even of those who learned *The Canon* by heart may have applied it effectively at all times and on all occasions; few may have meditated sufficiently to consider the soul-life of the patient they were called upon to help. But the life was there then, as it is here now. It could be read then, as it should be now. The entry to the infinite treasure-house of nature was not locked then, and it is not locked now. Indeed, the entry was not merely through one door, there was a portal of entry on every side. Doors so large as to be discernible from afar; doors so small that few could find them; but even through the smallest there was the same ability to enter the treasure-hall. Travelers in those days might fear imagined ogres, jinn, and terrifying guardians to counter talismans; but the keys of safety were everywhere in hand, for all these beings were amenable to caresses the caresses of a heart which approached them with reverence and affection, asking questions but never injuring; always treating everything within the treasury (for it is living) as gently as one should approach to watch a sleeping babe.

It is for us ourselves not to pass these things by. If we did nothing more than study the *materia medica* of those days to see what products were available, we should have ample material for thought, and become cognizant of the links between that age and this. The drugs are still cultivated, and still used in the East in the manner of the past, and the history of their names adds to our understanding of their uses. While it is true we can supply our needs through an order to the apothecary based on information imparted to us through various intermediaries, we may some day find that in doing so we have omitted to look inside the treasure-house. To go back to the old paths, watching nature and studying the uses of the living plants, is not to lose the definite therapeutic effects we seek. Far from it; and there is the added insight into that universal life which needs transference from the inexhaustible abundance of nature at large into the thirsting lack of the patient in particular. It would then be not simply as a "relaxation" from the exacting labors of the city that one would go abroad into the country-side. It would be for the purpose of retiring to watch, and meditate upon the manifestations of the quiet persistent surging life of creatures below the level of man, thereby to learn something of the secret through which the equilibrium of health is to be restored to the needy and also oneself—to receive from the fountains of life.

Dietetic Treatment

In these days, this form of treatment is increasingly to the fore. But whereas modern thought is in terms of food-values and the like, *The Canon* insists (and rightly) on the necessity for studying physiological and psychological incompatibilities in regard to each component of the diet, and for selecting the various articles of food according to their constitution, so that they shall be in harmony with the constitution of the patient.

Regiminal Treatment

The term "regimen" has a wide range. This has already been sufficiently indicated at the end of Part Three.[32] The consideration of the specific constitution of the patient, of his present state, and of the conditions which are likely to arise during the various successive phases of his illness, must pervade every detail of the prescription of the regimen, to ensure that the correspondences between the state and the various measures adopted shall throughout be as harmonious as possible.

In this way, the great importance of individual artistry in treatment is constantly insisted on, by contrast with the prevalent stereotyping of therapeutic methods, whether in regard to state regulated practice in its various branches, or in the provision of medical relief on a wholesale scale, or in the efforts to subject as much as possible to the output of team-work. The atmosphere thus created helps the student to realize that the last word has not been said when the clinician's discourse over the hospital bed is ended, and the protocols, and therapeutic orders have been set upon the bed sheet.

The following may be quoted here, from Bauer:[33]

> "It is true, there is a difference between the pure medical science and the art of its practical application at the patient's bedside. This art is somewhat more, indeed, than this application; it requires more than a complete knowledge of all scientific details; it is and will be always an art which never will be transformed into an exact science, as the complete understanding of one person's psychophysical machinery never will permit us to understand a second man's personality just as well by a pure analogy, because of the practically infinite variability of the individual constitution. The individual analysis must start always anew, and what science of the human constitution may help, is only to establish certain groups of more or less pronounced common characteristics . . . it will never replace entirely the doctor's art to . . . take the individual particularities of his patient into consideration . . . in constructing his diagnosis and in applying the fitted treatment."

The clinical handling of a case is guided from time to time by the experience which has been concentrated into aphorisms. Like many; ancient medical works, The Canon abounds in these also, and some of them will not doubt be found among the modern collections of aphorisms which are available. In this way, too, it may be true to say that the conduct of a modern case sometimes receives the personal guidance of the wisdom of the past.

Progress

Progress[34] is a relative term. The common error is to assume that it is an end in itself. Things which can be described as "up to date," or cast aside as "out of date," do not belong to the real basis of human life. The idea of progress is associated with the introduction of mechanical improvements of all kinds; with mass production of manufactured articles; with the standardization of existence. In the domain of medicine, it is more particularly associated with an increasing knowledge of concrete facts, with specific discoveries in etiology and treatment; and with a new nomenclature.

To illustrate the relative character of "progress" one may call to mind that many discoveries and inventions are simply actualizations of ideas previously current among thinkers, but perhaps not noticed at the time, or even repudiated or attacked as heretical. Further, as to the changes in nomenclature which occur as time goes on: because our language and idiom is different, many are apt to think the old statements were necessarily incorrect. In medieval books dealing with *materia medica*, they said for instance: "dissolved in vinegar, the action is so-and-so," whereas we say simply: acetum, action and uses: . . . In chemistry, they might say "fire produces YZ," whereas we says "on heating Z, the result is Y and X." In medical text-books there are innumerable diseases which are not mentioned in old works; and some diseases of the old books do not appear in modern ones. This is partly explained by the undoubted fact that we have diseases which once did not exist, whereas other conditions, very common in those days, certainly never occur now. The methods of teaching are different. In these days we convey information much more quickly and readily by diagrams, charts, tables, styles of print, not to mention experiments,.and moving-pictures. This fact does not prove that the learning of those days, acquired so laboriously, was faulty.

That which is called "progress" is also sometimes merely "fashion." The search for an elixir of life, for instance, has not ceased in the least. The gland therapy for restoring youth is perhaps the most conspicuous of modern variants of ancient research. Cupping and venesection were habitually used solely with the idea of "keeping fit" they have given place to the vogue of athletics and sport. New treatments for various conditions are introduced from time to time, and seem to be great advances because they are often conspicuously successful at first. How often do they not give place to still newer methods, and perhaps finally pass into entire oblivion? The fashion changes, and the old, is supplanted.

It will be suggested that knowledge is not simply "acquaintance with an assemblage of facts" and that facts in the aggregate do not suffice to constitute "truth."[35] There is a tendency to extol the acquisition of facts, as "adding to the sum of knowledge," and as being evidence of "progress." There are different forms of knowledge: human, angelic, divine. The perfection of knowledge is wisdom. There are different forms of truth: scientific, logical, moral, ontological, philosophical, theological, etc. But as to "Ultimate Truth," this is humanly unattainable, as may be illustrated by the accompanying diagram.

The observer and the thing observed are shown in plan, as being separated by a straight semi-transparent screen. The letters A to I represent the position of as many observers. For the purpose of illustration these are supposed to be of different nationalities and not necessarily acquainted with one another's language; they also belong to different periods of life (childhood, youth, etc.). The observer at A may be supposed only to be able to see the part of the object marked A; the observer at B. similarly, may only be able to see the part marked B. and so on. But even if any of the observers could see several parts, evidently there still remain some areas which are out of the range of vision of all persons, as marked K. L, M. No one can comprehend the whole, under the restrictions given.[36]

This conception may be applied to the interpretation of terms applied even to familiar objects. In studying The Canon, for instance, it is not enough to know the dictionary equivalent of an Arabic or Latin word, for the full meaning is not always adequately conveyed thereby. The word "*akhlat*" may be taken as an example. It is rendered humour, humour, body-fluid, juice. The impression conveyed by each equivalent varies according to ideas commonly associated with the word and the circumstances under which we first heard it. The conception of the word humour was necessarily different in the mind of the ancient Greek physician, of the Hindu sage. of the erudite Chinese, of the alchemist of the Middle Ages, of the characters in Shakespeare, of the modern laity, of the student of esotericism, and of the modern bio-chemist.

It has been said that we shall reach Truth by whatever road we take. But this is not so. There is really only one path which will take us there direct. All the others are devious and arduous, and in t he end only bring us to the confines of Truth. We may trace out every separate road as outlined for us by as many separate thinkers of the past or present; we may pursue the highway which modern science has opened out; we may decide also to study the tracks with which we are furnished by nature itself. But even after all these have been slowly and laboriously surveyed by spiritual insight, the best we can attain is but the fringe of Reality.

The Relation Between *The Canon* and Modern Thought

Considerations[37] are not wanting which entitle The Canon of Medicine of Avicenna to an esteemed position in modern thought. In the first place, there is the outstanding intellectual culture of the [Islamic] Empire—during the period of history to which Avicenna belongs. Secondly, in the case of much of his teaching, it may be said that the difference from ours is largely only that his speech is alien and is apt to be misunderstood. In these days, the great complexity of the language with which we express our scientific thought corresponds with the intricacy of the instruments wherewith facts are elicited. Thirdly, many of the advances of modern times offer the solutions to the very theorems and propositions of former times. Finally, ideas are to be found in his work which provide suggestions for useful research in the future.

The importance of idea over material achievement is not to be forgotten. The achievements of any age are subject to decay with the lapse of centuries but the ideas which gave rise to them remain living through all cycles. Therefore to propose a real place for Avicenna in modern thought is not to propose a return as it were to old architecture, or the costumes of long ago. It is rather to render accessible today the picture which he painted and so enable it to renew its still vital message. It is to play over again the music which he expressed and enable perhaps one or two to rejoice in it. And this without obscuring the issue by discussing nationality or schools of thought or evolution of ideas or technical methods.

If it appear to some a fault that the master appears to have used passages from other works and this without full acknowledgment, it should be remembered that after all a painter may use pigments which someone else has manufactured and is allowed even to employ other persons (usually pupils) to execute certain portions of his picture. Indeed, even after his decease, it is not improper that some may have been entrusted with the delicate task of touching up faded portions of the canvas which he bequeathed.

The place for Avicenna in modern thought is gained when it is agreed that he shall be viewed as one who entered this world entrusted with a mission independently to express for that age, by means of those various tools which he then found in it, the wisdom which is unchanging and impersonal. So also there is the need today that this same wisdom should be re-expressed for this age by means of the new data which lie to our hands.

The Intellectual Culture Contemporary with Avicenna

Carra de Vaux, in his monograph Avicenna[38] furnishes particularly striking comments, as follows:

"The more we investigate the enormous literary output of the [Islamic] empire and come into intimate appreciation of the master minds of the middle epoch and of antiquity, the more we become aware of their sincerity.

"We should, we think, offer our salutations to these great personalities of that day whose works and lives were equally encyclopedic.

"Our own times do not show more worthy figures; we complacently assume that there are no more worthy than ourselves because science, so greatly developed today, cannot be held all within one single head. That may be. But it is only right to admit that science has less unity and harmony today than formerly it had; that it is less pure than it was under the grand peripatetic discipline. Our attitude towards that is neither humble nor sincere.

"In these days we are concerned too much to have our name blazoned forth than to grasp a great extent of science. We are more anxious to uphold the profession than to have a passion for study; we seek titles and reputation rather than real know-ledge; and in order to appear more specialized than our ancestors wet expose ourselves to the judgment of posterity as having smaller minds and fettered souls."

As to the state of civilization in the western Saracen empire we have the very illuminating description of Ameer Ali,[39] "The Muslims covered the countries where they settled with networks of canals. To Spain they gave the system of irrigation by flood-gates, wheels and pumps. Whole tracts of land which now lie waste and barren were covered with olive groves, and the environs of Seville alone, under Muslim rule, contained several thousand oil factories. They introduced the staple products, rice, sugar, cotton, and nearly all the fine garden and orchard fruits, together with many less important plants, like ginger, saffron, myrrh, etc. They opened up the mines of copper, sulphur, mercury, and iron. They established the culture of silk, the manufacture of paper and other textile fabrics; of porcelain, earthenware, iron, steel, leather. The tapestries of Cordova, the woolen stuffs of Myrcia, the silks of Granada, Almeria, and Seville, the steal and gold work of Toledo, the paper of Salibah, were sought all over the world. The ports of Malaga, Carthage, Barcelona and Cadiz were vast commercial emporia for export and import. In the days of their prosperity, the Spanish Muslims maintained a merchant navy of more than a thousand ships. They had factories and representatives on the Danube. With Constantinople they maintained a great trade which ramified from the Black Sea, and the eastern shores of the Mediterranean into the interior of Asia, and reached the ports of India and China, and extended along the African coast as far as Madagascar.

> "In the midst of the tenth century, when Europe was about in the same condition that Caffraria is now, enlightened Moors, like Abul Cassem were writing treatises on the principles of trade and commerce. In order to supply an incentive to commercial enterprise, and to further the impulse to travel, geographical registers, gazetteers, and itineraries were published under the authority of the government, containing minute descriptions of the places to which they related, with particulars of the routes and other necessary matters. Travelers like Ibn Battuta visited foreign lands in quest of information, and wrote voluminous works on the people of those countries, on their fauna and flora, their mineral products, their climate and physical features, with astonishing perspicacity and keenness of observation.
>
> "The love of learning and arts was by no means confined to one sex. The culture and education of the women proceeded on parallel lines with that of the men and women were as keen in the pursuit of literature and as devoted to science as men. They had their own colleges;[40] they studied medicine and jurisprudence, lectured on rhetoric, ethics, and belles-lettres and participated with the stronger sex in the glories of a splendid civilization. The wives and daughters of magnates and sovereigns spent their substance in founding colleges and endowing universities, in establishing hospitals for the sick, refuges for the homeless, the orphan and the widow."

Cordova was the most celebrated western university of the Empire at the time of Avicenna. This is well known as an instance of the high degree of culture of the day. Ameer Ali speaks of "that wonderful kingdom of Cordova, which was the marvel of the Middle Ages, and which when all Europe was plunged in barbaric ignorance and strife alone held the torch of learning and civilization bright and shining before the western world."[41] The greatness of the city is indicated by its population which is given by Haeser[42] as 300,000, and by Campbell[43] as one million; and by the library of "about 200,000" volumes.

To see the city today, traversed as it can be from wall to wall, within half an hour on foot, and to read of an extent of "twenty-four miles one way and six in the other"[44] shows that the word "kingdom" conveys a truer idea of its greatness. To read of "innumerable libraries, 3,800 mosques, 60,000 palaces and mansions, 200,000 houses inhabited by the common people, 3700 baths, 80,000 shops, besides hostels and caravanserais" is to wonder how so much can have come to be now represented by so little ("every dwelling-place, even if it has been blessed ever so long, will one day become a prey."[45] Nevertheless, the "grand mosque" alone, which is still at any rate externally intact (and interiorly is still surely one of the wonders of the world despite its mutilation) stands sponsor for the rest; and no doubt many of the existing imposing buildings—now devoted to very different uses—stand for the palaces and mansions. As to the literary treasures, these have been traced at least in part from Spain to Fez, as shown by Horne,[46] with the Roud El Qartas as his authority; and he then points to years of pilfering from the library of the great mosque of El Karouiyan at Fez, as having scattered these works forever.

A study of the street names, and even the place names and current dialect in "Moorish Spain" today also confirms the story of past greatness. But the mystical knowledge displayed in the dispositions of the decorative designs and their poetic inscriptions on the walls of the Alhambra halls, state-rooms, and private apartments can leave no doubt of unsurpassed artistic power where every sense impression was deliberately drawn on. Lights and shadows and colors changing with the hours of the day; musical effects of simultaneous diversity of disposition of flowing water; perfumes; courting of the prevailing breezes; interior architectural form; and furnishings, animate and manufactured—all these were combined for the achievement of a perfect representation of (divine, over and above human) beauty.

Among the Chinese? The bearing of Chinese philosophical thought on the subject of Avicenna lies in the fact that we here meet with a notable example of intimacy of relation between world conception and medicine. The writings which are so carefully studied today by so many sinologists were extant at the time of Avicenna, and are still held in the highest esteem by Chinese thinkers. The modern Chinese philosopher is supposed to say to the westerner, "What is the reason for which you deem yourselves our betters? Have you excelled us in arts or letters?

Have our thinkers been less profound than yours? Has our civilization been less elaborate, less complicated, less refined than yours? Why, when you lived in caves and clothed yourselves with skins, we were a cultured people . . . ."[47]

The attitude towards western learning so displayed may be blamed by many, but is certainly praised by those who have studied the philosophy most deeply. As long ago as 1876 we read conclusive evidence.[48] If some students discuss their philosophy with a certain cynicism,[49] others[50] see into the justice of their conceptions. As Caruso remarks: "We need not be blind to the many errors and absurdities of the ancient occultism to understand and grant the truth that underlies its system."[51] These words are exactly applicable to *The Canon of Medicine* of Avicenna.

The Nature of the Knowledge Presented by *The Canon*

The Canon is a precis and not a sum-total of Avicenna's knowledge. Numerous passages occur in *The Canon* which show that this is the case, that it is a series of notes or skeleton outlines of thought not too lengthy to be memorized by his students[52] much as they would memorize the Quran. Thus, "to the full extent necessary, and yet with apt brevity,"[53] "do not place in medicine what does not belong to it,"[54] "having discussed the equable temperaments sufficiently,"[55] "I purposely omit reference to certain other problems relative to the fluids of the body just as much as is necessary to enable you to practice medicine intelligently."[56] Many passages also refer to others of his own works for further details, to avoid confusing the purely medical issue of *The Canon*. These philosophical works are gradually becoming more widely known.

"Generally speaking, the saying of the saints and sages are terse, presenting only the germs of truth; these are developed by later teachers and then expanded and added to. We must see to it, however, that we get at the original meaning of the saints and sages."[57]

"Books are only words and the valuable part of words is the thought therein contained. That thought has a certain bias, which cannot be conveyed in words, yet the world values words as being the; essence of books. But though the world values them, they are not of value; as that sense in which the world values them is not the sense in which they are valuable."[58]

To say that a work is the product of the age in which an author lives is certainly often an error, for it is to confuse the person's insight with the tools (the language at his command) available to express himself with.

Similarly to work out the relation between a literary work and the religious belief of the author, as for instance to show the relation between Islamic science and the Quran carries the same fallacy with it. The Prophet said, "Every soul when born is a faithful follower; it is afterwards that he becomes unfaithful"—which is to say that the form of religious belief is a secondary implantation, whereas the spirit of a sincere life can be traced to the original being.

Avicenna's medicine, like Indian medicine, has been traced to the Greek system. But it has been proved that the great works of *Charaka* and *Susruta* were available in Arabic, under the title of *Kitab shawshura al-Hindi*, from the 7th century.[59] Similarly, the view that the Chinese borrowed their philosophy of the five elements from the Turks has been sufficiently disposed of by Forke.[60] It is beside the purpose of this treatise to take up such questions.

The common notion that progress or stagnation in secular knowledge has a causal relationship with a certain religion is typically voiced in his address on "*Medicine and the Church*" by Sir Farquhar Buzzard.[61] The comment to make is: "*post hoc sed non propter hoc*." The advances in the science of medicine, as in all other sciences, are surely a part of the divine plan for mankind whereas the collateral abandonment of religious fundamentals remains a human responsibility.

The word "canon" (*qanun*): equivalent words: code of laws; series of principles; tao.[62] Principle is defined as "something antecedent, which exercises a real positive influence upon the consequent" = causes (four kinds, Avicenna) = reasons.

In view of this it is clear that *The Canon* is not properly to be regarded as an "encyclopedia" of the knowledge of the time, or to be contrasted, for instance, with the now classical "*Osler*."

The word "knowledge": knowledge is not simply an assemblage of "facts" nor is it to be made synonymous with "truth"—certainly not Absolute Truth, of which all human knowledge falls short although one single word is capable of containing or implying all knowledge, as in mathematics a single term may be equated with an infinite number of terms summed together. But even the mathematical sciences can only afford approximate truth.[63] We may recall the words, "If he attain to all knowledge, he is far off still."[64]

Facts, as St. Thomas[65] explains, are what our intellect regards as external objects—and as we judge of them only in terms of our sense organs—these objects may be different. God knows them as they are. Our intellect depends on our imagination and that depends on our senses. Our senses only convey discrete fragments which we gather into one continuous impression regardless of intervening points." We live as it were in a network only the nodes of which are evident to the senses.

Mystical Insight

There is a distinction between knowledge gained in the ordinary manner and that gained by "mystical insight" (*kashf*). The writer of *Gulshan-i-raz's*[66] advises his readers to follow this, saying:

> Straightway lift yourself above time and space,
> Quit the world and be yourself a world for yourself.
> And
>
> The moment we are enlightened within
> We go beyond the voidness of a world confronting us.
> —Seng-ts'an, quoted by Susuki.[67]

As this "opens up all of a sudden a world hitherto undreamed of, it is an abrupt and discrete leaping from one plane of thought to another."[68]

> Real science is seeing the fire directly,
> Not mere talk, inferring the fire from the smoke.
> Your scientific proofs are more offensive to the wise
> Than the urine and breath whence a physician infers.[69]

"Man looks at the surface of the ocean. Yet he is so small that he cannot even be compared to one of its drops, limited as he is in intellect and in his knowledge. It is only to those who, having just touched creation, bow to God, forgetting their limited self, that God has remained. These through whom God has spoken are the only beings who have been able to give any truth to the world."[70]

"The mind is not like a horizontal door which haste be made larger by force. You must clear away the obstructions arising from creaturely desire and then it will be pure and clear with no limit to its knowledge. Heng Ch'u said, 'When the mind is enlarged it can enter into everything throughout the universe.' He who praises God knows about Him."[71]

This attitude towards nature is to be claimed for Avicenna on the plain evidence of his other writings including the *al-Najat* which appropriately appears in the Arabic version of *The Canon* printed at Rome in 1593 and of the Libellus on the powers of the hearts and is included in the Latin edition of *The Canon*, 1595.[72]

The acquisition of knowledge by this process demands nothing more than a keen observation of the life around us and was as much within his reach as ours. Such knowledge is not too restricted to one period of history, one language, or to one or two universities. And if it should seem that because our civilization is so different his opportunities were much less, we may pause to reflect that the difference between our age and his is chiefly one of mechanical appurtenances and phraseology; and that even to this day we need not travel far (i.e., the old streets of Cordova and Granada or more definitely, to northern Africa) to see much the same sort of scenery as he was accustomed to, much the same sort of life as is drawn in the 1001 Nights. In any case, what is human life, at bottom, but a matter of buying and selling, receiving and giving, seizing and relinquishing, constructing and demolishing, acquiring learning and losing it, seeking power and breaking it, bidding and forbidding, giving in marriage and seeking to obtain in marriage, birth and death.

The significant phrase "seeing into one's own nature,"[73] in which most admirable work occur many passages by way of explanation) gives a graphic description of that which gives Avicenna his superiority. *The Canon* is simply the medical garb in which the one Truth is expounded. It is for us also to perceive it in whatever idiom it might be described—western, eastern, Islamic, Confucian or Buddhist, for example.

It would then seem as if the mind were now able to float as it were round all the concepts the human being has ever given to the world, or round all the most familiar events of one's daily life, and perceive clearly that which can never be set forth in words. We should then also quote the words."[74] I perceive of it that it is something, but what it is I cannot perceive. Only it seems if I could conceive it, I should comprehend all truths.

Further than this, to find that some of the statements in *The Canon* are certainly erroneous and that modern investigations have placed us at an infinitely greater advantage, does not invalidate the work as a whole. Its possibilities for suggesting thoughts of real value today are more realized the more one reads between the lines, and the present treatise does not claim to exhaust them.

"Let not the authority of the writer offend thee, whether he be of title or great learning, but let the love or pure truth entice thee to read."[75]

Insight into eternal truths. A person may: (1) glimpse them; (2) understand them moderately; (3) understand them fairly thoroughly. But in describing them to another, he may explain them: (i) imperfectly (no one can explain them properly!); (ii) inadequately or incompletely; (iii) wrongly because of: (a) imperfect education; (b) educational bias; (c) religious or anti-religious bias; (d) inherently erroneous methods of thought; (e) restriction to logic. Such truths, again, may be denied by persons being told of them, for because in their turn they misunderstand, or understand only in part, either through careless attention, and (a) to (e).

Insight Versus Intuitional Knowledge

A note should here be made that the term "insight" as used here bears a rather different meaning to that pertaining to the term "intuitive knowledge," which St. Thomas[76] ascribes solely to the angelic mind, and defines as "the attainment of the truth of a thing at a single glance without the aid of reasoning."[77] On the other hand this mode of perceiving truths need not be disallowed a rudimentary commencement among the powers of the human soul, just as the "brute" mind must be allowed to contain rudiments of those high mental capacities which characterize the human being. Throughout all orders of creation, the lower are endowed with the scaffolding for the manifestation of successively more exalted capacities of the higher.

The Basic Difference between The Canon and Modern Medicine

The Canon treats of:

I. Speculative Medicine
   Certain fundamental principles (cosmology, psychology, metaphysics)

II. Practical Medicine
   A. Application of Speculative Medicine to the study of (i) health; (ii) disease (tendency, predisposition, threshold stage, declared disease; (iii) cessation of life.
   B. Actual treatment of "disease" by: (i) regimen, (ii) drugs, (iii) operative interference.

Modern Medicine consists of:

A. Principles of Medicine: The application of the facts of chemistry, physics, anatomy, biology to the systematic description of innumerable "diseases" classified as far as possible on the basis of the microbic theory; symptomatology; etiology; diagnosis.

B. Practice of Medicine
   i) Laboratory work

ii) Therapeutics, Pharmacology and Dietetics
iii) Surgery
iv) Gynecology and Obstetrics
v) States of Medicine: Hygiene in all its ranches
vi) Psychological Medicine: Treatment of insanity
vii)Legal medicine, etc.

Modern medicine is based on the conception of the universe as a conglomeration of dead matter out of which, by some unexplainable process, life may become evolved in forms. To Avicenna the whole of the universe is the manifestation of a universal principle of life, acting through the instrumentality of forms. Or, again, in modern medicine, the forms are the source of life; to Avicenna they are the product of life. Space itself is an aspect of the one life.[78]

In this way the difference between Avicenna's conception of "principles," and that of modern medicine is easily shown. To the school boy "science" would consist of (a) bookwork and (b) laboratory work which his teachers would insist is the basis of (a). Similarly, the medical curriculum begins with lectures, although these are more and more inclined to become laboratory demonstrations; and goes on to laboratory and hospital work.

In short, Avicenna's medicine, and all ancient and traditional medicine, is intimately bound up with philosophy, to wit, that of human nature—a philosophy which proves to be virtually identical with "modern scholastic philosophy," no doubt partly because the Quranic account of the origin of the human being tallies with the Christian.

Modern medicine, on the other hand, assuming the title and rank of a positive science, emphatically discards and excludes it. Hence we read: "the physiologist" (said Burdon Sanderson) "can pursue philosophy if he has a turn for it, but must understand that the moment he enters the field of philosophy he leaves his tools behind him." For "it is unfortunate that the limitations of scientific thought were often ignored by men of science in their writings . . . the result diverts those who know, but befogs the unsuspicious reader who will probably put the blame on his intelligence."[79]

"According to positivism, science cannot be as Aristotle conceived it, the knowledge of things through their ultimate causes, since material and formal causes are unknowable, final causes are illusions, and efficient causes are simply invariable antecedents, while metaphysics under any form is illegitimate."[80] Or, expressed more boldly, "philosophy" is considered to be the exact antithesis of the truth which modern medicine gives us, and is therefore inherently inadmissible to medicine.

The ignorance which accounts for this attitude is only met by insisting on proper definitions of terms. The following apply here:

Philosophy is "the science which is concerned with first causes and principles; it is the profound knowledge of the universal order, and the duties which that order imposes on the human being.[81]

Again, philosophy is the true perception and understanding of cause and effect. Metaphysics is "that portion of philosophy which treats of the most general and fundamental principles underlying all reality and all knowledge."[82] Psychology is "the science which treats of the soul and its operations" and, therefore, clearly, must be the real foundation of medicine.

It is in modern scholastic philosophy that the student finds ample exposure of the fallacy in positivism and its cognates, enabling him to detect the difference between false and true, expressed with enough force of logic to satisfy the most meticulous. This queen of all the sciences amply proves positivist science (including medicine) to be incomplete knowledge when taken alone. The knowledge of movement or change must be supplemented by mathematical and metaphysical viewpoints.[83] Such men as Albertus Magnus and Roger Bacon were convinced of the necessity of linking the sciences with philosophy.[84]

When medicine has in this way become ennobled it reaches its highest degree of perfection, in that it penetrates to the very depths of reality,85 admitting this knowledge to need, even then, a further complement to make it complete-namely, knowledge in relation to God ("Christian wisdom").

> *"Sapientia est scientia qua considerat causas primas et universales causas. Sapientia causas primas omnium causarum considerat."86 "Ille qui cognoscit causam altissimam simpliciter, qua est Deus dicitur sapiens simpliciter, in quantum per regulas divinas omnia potest judicare et ordinare."*[87] *"Non acquiritur studio humano, sed est deursum scendens."*[88] *"Cum homo per res creatas Deum cognoscit, magis videtur hoc perti nere ad scientiam, ad quam perti net formaliter, qu am ad sapientiam ad qu am pertinet materialiter: et e converso cum secundum res divinas judicamus de rebus creatis, magis hoc ad sapientiam quam ad scientiam pertinet."*[89]

As St. Thomas said in his day, "they think that nothing exists besides visible creatures." [N.B.:"Creatures" are (a) animate; and (b) inanimate]. "They think that things proceed not by the divine will but by natural necessity."[90] So even in those days time and fortune were expended on researches which sound philosophy would have shown to be inherently futile.

We may reflect for instance on the reiterated search for a location of the soul, which the pioneer anatomists prosecuted, and also on the commonly repeated announcement to successive students of anatomy that the pineal gland is now no longer regarded as the site of the soul. There is the sub-conscious suggestion to the student that scientific research has effectively disposed of the medieval belief in the soul, whereas history only proves that the revolt against the precise teachings of the Council of Trent necessarily came to naught.[91] The very definition of "soul" which this council laid down makes a search for its location ludicrous.

Special Differences Between The Canon and Modern Medicine

Conceptions Known to Avicenna Not Now Recognized

There are four main conceptions belonging to *The Canon*, but not recognized by modern medicine. To use St. Thomas' words, they can be shown to be "not impossible";[92] that is, the discoveries of modern science do not abrogate them.

These conceptions are relative to: (1) the nature of the human being as a whole; (2) the constitution; (3) the "breath"; (4) the "elements." Each of these is dealt with in some detail under the corresponding sections of *The Canon*, but some of the salient points are suitably referred to at this stage.

The varieties of views on conception of the nature of the human being as a whole, which people in every country and race exhibit both in conversation and in literature, numerous though they are, are capable of classification under one of three headings: (1) The Platonic view—regards the human being as "soul within a body," while admitting "soul" to be indefinable, and beyond the power of location. This view, widely supposed to be "Christian," is well known as "pagan" to students of folklore. (2) The scientific or rationalistic and modern view—takes the physical body as the fundamental, seeing in it the outcome of known or at least knowable forces. The facts of anatomy, physiology, etc., convey their own inevitable conclusions. This view makes its immediate appeal. From the first lesson the pupil is able to feel a grasp of some tangible knowledge, whereas the alternative third view entails a long study before the intricacies of abstract philosophy can be mastered. The difference between experience and "poring over books" is only too obvious. The possibility of interweaving the two methods is not on the horizon.

In its answer to "religion," this scientific view has no objection to raise to its votaries retaining a private belief in the Platonic view, if their temperament demands it. But this "pious belief" must not be allowed to vitiate procedure when scientific research is undertaken.

This modern conception regards the body as an aggregate of "spare parts" which are "assembled" well, or ill; can be repaired, or remedied. According as the assembling is good or bad, and, according to the "fuel," so is there health, or susceptibility to infection by organisms. The kind of assembling is a matter partly heredity and partly of environment.

The following remarks in a review on a recent article in Science.[93] They present the idea in technical language:

> "Physiology finds the organism to be a nexus of physicochemical determination; differing only from non-living systems in its complexity. . . . Speaking of freewill, one argument against indeterminism is that the energy balance sheet of a man shows us there is no creation of energy within the body. To assume will-power we conflict with Newton's first law. . . . The ultra microscope alone suggests indeterminism, and even this may be only because we do not know enough about Brownian movement, etc. Protoplasm is a heterogeneous system. In heredity sub-microscopical units determine the details of inheritance—but an event originating in an ultra-microscopic particle can spread to the whole cell or organism. On this view, a human action appearing entirely spontaneous and voluntary to the actor and spectator would exhibit itself as a succession of mechanically determined events capable of study and prediction in all its microscopic details. But traced inward it would ultimately resolve itself into certain ultramicroscopic events in the interior of the nerve-cell." But "even the freedom of the ultra-microscopic particle may be no more than a subtler kind of determinism beyond the reach of present analysis."[94]

It may be noted, in passing, that the doctrine of vitalism is really only another form of rationalism, as will appear when the scholastic doctrine is duly investigated.

The third view—scholastic, Thomistic-presented by modern scholastic philosophy has the Aristotelian basis. Its soundness is best appreciated by careful study prolonged until the prevalent inadequate and illogical conceptions of the universe are clearly exposed. Briefly, the view is expressed in the words: "the human being is a material body vivified by a life-principle, the two together constituting the rational human soul." As St. Thomas says, "It is not my soul that thinks, or my body that eats, but 'I' that do both."[95] In other words, again: The body and "soul" form one complete whole—one "single being."[96]

It is this view which underlies the whole *Canon*, and is expounded in connection with the corresponding parts of the text. It is this view that makes the ancient work fall in line with the most "modern." Its consequences are far-reaching. The external configuration of the body, including the physiognomy, is a reflection of the functional capacity of the internal organs and general make-up of the individual. The character, talents, physical form, shape of individual features, general development, and indeed every detail of the physique, length of limbs, of fingers, cutaneous markings, contour of the eyes and ears, etc., ark all part and parcel with the functional conformations of the viscera, and the mental characters; a study of the visible will inform of the nature of the internal conformation.[97]

The idea that from a study of external features and general habit one should deduce conclusions as to functional capacities[98] is generally opposed by academic medicine; as is voiced by F. Muller when he says, "We must steadfastly avoid drawing any far-reaching conclusions about the functional behavior of the organism from a study of the external characters of the body."[99]

While it may be urged that the external features are usually misread, it may also be admitted that even the customary "physical examination" of a patient does not yield uniform results when practiced, as it necessarily is, by persons of varying talent. Surely, the remedy is to exert greater care. We may, for instance, observe how a skilled weaver will detect the site of a flaw in the "set-up" of a loom by a mere glance, whereas a novice discovers it only after laborious search.

On the other hand, the biochemical tests for functional capacity of organs—so much the vogue and so much exploited, and so duly impressive on patients and their friends—are clearly inadequate in the light of the scholastic doctrine. It is true that the attempt to force the intangible to yield to mathematical formula rules and weights and measures (as, for instance, in blood-cholesterol analysis is sincere enough, to judge by the time, energy and money expended so freely).

But what is to be the verdict once it is realized that the anatomical organs are not functionally discrete or amenable to distinctive "specific" tests? A just appreciation of the intimacy of relation inherent in the conception of the human being insisted on here suffices to show the futility of those labors and studies whether made upon man or upon the various orders of animals taken instead.

More than this, there is the conception that the internal organs belong to one another beyond the anatomical limits. The heart, to anatomy, is a circumscribed organ; to Avicenna it is part of a force occupying the whole body. "The human heart is both corporeal and incorporeal."[100] So, again, the liver is simply a visible portion of a "liver" whose operation pervades the whole body.[101] Or to combine modern with ancient knowledge, the physical heart, the arterial vessels, and the sympathetic nervous system, including the connections between this and the sensorium and that which corresponds to the "sensitive soul" in its emotional aspect, for instance—all this is one great composite; and its state is also reflected in many subtle indications which offer themselves to the keen observer of the patient.

The modern research on diseases of the brain and insanity is based on the assumption that the material brain is the source of all nervous activities, which are correlated with definite biochemical, physicochemical and even structural changes in brain substance. Mental disease is the outcome of similar changes The Platonists would consider mental disease as apart from the "soul." The Thomistic view leads to much more subtle conclusions, capable of lasting influence.

The Doctrine of "The Constitution"

The term "constitution" conveys different ideas to different minds. The laity regard the term as synonymous with "temperament" or "make-up," at least in part, and consider a description of a patient as haying a nervous temperament, a delicate constitution, etc., quite adequate. With this goes the conviction among the lay that the medical curriculum leaves the graduate fully able to " understand his constitution" whereas in actual fact the subject is never discussed. The study of physique is quite superficial and is admittedly made solely to establish a diagnosis of specific "diseases." Hence the term, in conversation, is actually nothing more than platitudes.

To modern medicine, regarding the body as corporeal, constitution is a matter of physique, resistance to disease, mode of reaction to various stimuli (including psychic stimuli). Classifications of varieties of constitution on this basis are afforded by various writers in all countries —i.e., a classification into athletic, leptosomic and dysplastic; into arthritic, endocrine, lymphatic, asthenic, infantilistic, chlorotic, etc. (current medical journals).

In *The Canon*, Avicenna establishes "constitution" in terms of humours, temperaments (hot, cold, dry, moist) and "elements" (whose proportions are set. for every individual). If we go further, and apply to this term the method which Rumi,[102] the great Persian sage demanded of students of the Quran, we shall not regard a patient's constitution as understood until we have studied the matter much more intimately.

> Know the words of the Quran are simple,
> But within the outward sense is an inner secret one.
> Beneath that secret meaning is a third,
> Whereat the highest wit is dumbfounded.
> The fourth meaning has been seen by none
> Save God, the Incomparable and All-sufficient.
> Thus they go on, even to seven meanings, one by one,
> According to the saying of the Prophet, without doubt.

"I know," said Tawaddud, the lady most learned, "the sublime Quran by heart and have read it according to the seven, the ten, and the fourteen modes."[103]

Therefore, to draw a lesson for our study out of these indications, we shall see that the aim in view is to formulate a person's constitution out of a number of components, none of which must be omitted from the series. To express the whole picture many modern aspects must be studied—histological, biochemical, psychological, without neglecting factors (metaphysical, etc.) accepted by the ancients but almost forgotten today. For instance, the past events in the ancestral history of the patient must be included and all the factors coming into play even from the time of quickening may not be overlooked.

The insight afforded by the true conception of the nature of the human being in this way leads us on to an understanding of individual constitutions which should be amply satisfactory.

The Doctrine of "The Breath"

This subject is discussed in the course of the text.[104] The term "breath" found in Eastern writings is taken as the exact equivalent of Avicenna's conception, and is understood properly only when the "elements" are understood.[105]

Equivalent terms: life-principle; *hayat*; the breath of life; *virtus vitalis*; *spiritus*; vitality; *Hu* (in Persian mysticism; Hu in Chinese is not the exact equivalent although being used more for the act of expiration unless there is a mystical sense attached to the term); *Ch'i; nafas* (also used for "soul," "individuality").

It may be conceded that many of these words are used synonymously with much confusion in consequence. Thus the old doctrine of vitalism—

supported by vitalists—is not the antithesis of, but strictly speaking, another form of rationalism. In Paracelsus we read "the first matter of the elements is nothing else than life. The soul of the elements is the life of all created things. . . . There is again a difference between the soul and the life. Fire if it lives, burns. But if it be in its soul, that is; in its element, it lacks all power of burning."[106] Errors of this kind are avoided by a careful study of the scholastic philosophy.

The Doctrine of "The Elements"

This is fully entered into at the end of the corresponding chapter in the translation.[107] The conception of the universe in terms of four, or five, elements has been found among all peoples. To argue in favor of the doctrine almost compels an attempt at harmonization of its different forms (Aristotelian, Indian, Persian, Chinese, for instance). Suppose a number of people each set out to paint one certain landscape; that each is of different nationality; that each is restricted to a certain limited number of pigments; that each is a true artist. The final picture presented by each will be striking and inspiring. But it would be out of place to begin and compare stick with stick and stone with stone. If we understand, we shall learn from each, The modern futurist may excite ridicule in lets attempts to depict a landscape in terms of psychic forces, which he claims to discern, but to the mind of a student his work would have a different effect. These varying forms of one conception are amenable to intelligent understanding.[108]

Carus writes, "An explanation of the universe which derives all distinctions between things, conditions, relations, etc., from differences of mixture must have appeared very plausible to the ancient sages . . . even today Western scientists of reputation attempt to explain the universe as a congeries of force-centers, acting either by attraction or repulsion in analogy to positive and negative electricity. On the ground of this fact the educated Chinese insist with more than a mere semblance of truth that the underlying idea of the Chinese world conception is fully borne out and justified by the results of Western science."[109] Elsewhere the intimacy, in fact unity, between this philosophy and everyday life is referred to as the justification for so often quoting Chinese thought in expounding Avicenna.[110]

Conceptions Known to Modern Medicine; but Not to Avicenna

Among the most important of these are: (1) the anatomy of the circulation of the blood. (2) the rate of that circulation. (3) The details found in The Canon's anatomy; the microscopic anatomy; such complexities as form the theme of Bayliss' Physiology. These details might be expressed as those of "the mechanics of the body." (4) Interactions in the tissues: chemical and cellular metabolism. (5) In pathology: the microbic theory; the endless and always increasing number of "diseases"; the laboratory diagnosis of dysfunction of organs; (albuminuria was, of course, unknown); symptoms as evidences of disordered reflexes. (6) In treatment: the use of antisera and specific anti-substances of organisms; hypodermic medication; complex drug treatment has passed out of vogue; surgery.

Considerations which suggest that these instances of ignorance are not as grave as is supposed, and do not invalidate the standing of ancient medicine in regard to actual practice.

Circulation of a kind was propounded in the case of the "breath," the elements, and the body-fluids, though not along anatomical channels. The Chinese recognized a process of "revolution," a succession of cyclical changes an ebb and flow. Indeed, it is suggested in *Duhalde*[111] that the Chinese knew of the circulation of the blood itself some hundred years BC.

Wieger,[112] discussing whether the Chinese knew of the circulation of the blood twenty centuries before Harvey or not, decides truly that "their knowledge of the circulation of the blood in the human microcosm was intuitive, not experimental, conjectured in imitation of the circulation of the vital principle in the universal microcosm, in which they believed. They guessed the fact, and they never verified it. . . . During more than twenty centuries, the how of the guessed circulation never worried their mind. The yin-yang circulates in a ring, the five agents do the same, the blood the same. That is all . . ." But if a doctrine which is common to Taoism and esotericism [that of microcosm and macrocosm] is allowed to be valid, the words "intuitive knowledge" cannot be made synonymous with "conjecture," "guess."

The rapidity of the changes was certainly not realized. The Chinese apparently believed that the circulation was completed only fifty times in one day. There is however room for fallacious.

Lest there should be over-satisfaction with ourselves, it may be suggested that the rapidity of the movement of the lymph was not realized before about 1908, and is perhaps not fully realized by many practitioners today; the rapidity of passage of food-materials down the small intestine was not known until the advent of the "bismuth" meal. The circulation of nerve-impulses is not yet admitted.

The capillaries of the liver are referred to[113] in the body in general.[114] True, what Avicenna calls capillaries are larger than those we see with the microscope. But he knew that the blood passes from large trunks into the liver, traverses "capillaries" in the liver, and re-emerges by large trunks.

Interactions in the tissues were conceived of as taking place with an ebb and a flow (which is correct); lymph exudes into the tissue-spaces. Interactions take a considerable time (true). Digestion goes on within the blood-vessels in various parts of the body.

Fermentation was the counterpart of bacterial growth as we know it. The term is used sufficiently specifically in the text.[115] Diseases were regarded chiefly as parts of a process; and there were but few processes (which is quite true: nine processes).116 Urinalysis was carried out in order to assess the functional state of the liver.[117]

Modern medicine claims its title to superiority by its successes, and judges the medicine of the past by its failures. But what would the judgment be if this method were reversed? Suppose we accepted the verdict of those among the laity (who are not so few) who are dissatisfied with their experiences of orthodox medicine and have turned to the "unqualified" of one kind or another, or those of other countries who prefer their native doctors still, or even those Europeans who have experienced triumphant success from native doctors, aver modern methods had failed? After all the ancient medicine is still practiced from Cairo to Calcutta, and a medicine not very different holds sway through the Far East. The late Sir Charles Pardy Lukis[118] is quoted as saying "Many of the empirical methods of treatment adopted by *hakims* are of the greatest value, and there is no doubt whatever that their ancestors, ages ago, knew many things which are nowadays being brought forward as new discoveries.[119]

Drug-treatment

The complexity of prescriptions of former times has given place to simple and short ones, and the tendency is to discard them altogether. But the reasons for the ancient method are given in the Canon, and Avicenna's choice of remedies depended on a careful consideration of the constitution of the remedies, as well as of the patient and his idiosyncrasies. Thus, certain ingredients would be allowed or disallowed in a given standard confection according to the nature of the particular patient. " The presence or absence, and the amount, of *nardus*, ginger, fennel-seed, anise, piper, *cyperus rotundus*, must be according to the season, and the age of the patient.[120]

F. Hartmann[121] describes the accuracy of native diagnosis[122] as "disconcerting," and describes certain forms of treatment (auto-chemotherapy, Bier treatment) as being practiced in a manner only different in outward appearance from the technique which we pride ourselves as being absolutely the "latest." "No wonder," he says, "that the Chinese are proud of their art, considering how long they have known that which we have only recently discovered." (These words can be fully endorsed, if only from a study of the Chinese classic on the pulse, Wan K'an t'ang, 80 volumes, discussed under the heading "*The Pulse*" in the present treatise.[123] Among other ancient Chinese medical works-first seen by the present writer in the very extensive collection in the Library of McGill University-reference may be made to the astonishing accuracy of representations of medicinal and other plants, and the almost dramatic representations of various diseases states in the *I tsung chin ch'un* by Hung Chou, extant in Avicenna's time. This work was reprinted between 1904 and 1924 and an older edition is in the Library of the *School of Oriental Studies*).

The cynical mind cannot be upheld which passes off the reputed successes during the Middle Ages as coincidences, and overlooks the modern crowded out-patient departments as evidences of the limitations of our current therapy and theory; nor can the skeptic be much noticed who denies miraculous cures rather than admit scientific theories to be in any sense inadequate.

Nevertheless, it is obvious that the principles of *The Canon* could not be taught over a hospital bed or in the out-patient department. It is true that they cannot cater for the wholesale requirements of the hospital or clinic. It should be clear to the candid that our modern technique does not avail for 100 per cent of cases; for those who do not benefit at least an experiment with other systems of treatment should not be denied. If the fault is laid at the feet of over-strenuous routine work, the more leisured may yet find an advantage in a system which puts the details of a person's constitution in all its aspects into the forefront, where there is no question of teaching it either to classes or even to possibly indifferent individuals. The words of Paracelsus may be recalled, where he says: a the doctor who loves his art does not undertake twenty cases but five, knowing that no one person can conscientiously treat more than a certain number. No one person could ever make the whole world sound."

Knowledge Common to Avicenna and Modern Medicine

A perusal of the text of The Canon will show many passages which apply quite well, without explanation, in these days. Thus, the following may be specified: the close relation between emotions and physiological states (shown to be even closer than modern research has realized); the classification of people into sanguine, phlegmatic, bilious, saturnine, frigid, "hot"; the physiology of sleep; and how posture may remedy insomnia.

Choice of Location for Dwellings

Health resorts. Climactic influences on health and illness- Plethoric maladies. Dietetics. Hydrotherapy. Regiminal treatment. The uses of counter-irritation. Bier treatment. The introduction of remedies into the urethra. The use of vaginal tampons. The use of anesthetics by the mouth (medicated wines: scopolamine). Testing the strength of a drug by animal experiment. The treatment of insanity by malaria.[124]

No doubt the great difference between the ancient and modern is one of outlook, which accounts for the difference of topic. That which appeared interesting and even important in those days is passed over by modern physiology and pathology. Each century has its own interests. The mistake made is to suppose that the older interests were "wrong," "incorrect," "useless"; and to label them as "out of date." True, fashions of all kinds come to be out of date, but the epithets "right," "wrong" do not apply. The more carefully we observe modern science the more evident does it become that just its terminology and subject of conversation is different Things are seen from new angles, and things only surmised at then are amenable to tangible description now.

In fact, there occur moments, even at this day, when suggestive thoughts might be drawn from The Canon, to help in studying the individual, tedious, or baffling case, especially where the practice is far distant from the laboratories and appliances of modern medicine.

Of Interest to the Scholar

The present translation is based on the Latin versions published at Venice in 1608 and 1595, supported by a study of the Arabic edition printed at Rome in 1593 and the Bulaq edition.

It is true that as E. G. Browne pointed out, "The Latin Qanun swarms with barbarous words which are not merely transcriptions, but in many cases almost unrecognizable mistranscriptions of Arabic originals,"[125] and that Hirschberg and Lippert[126] regard the Latin as almost unintelligible, though they admit the "slavish adherence" of the Latin to the Arabic. Campbell[127] states that there was a "society of translators" at Toledo, about 1130 A.D., "whose method of translating from Arabic to Latin was to put the Latin equivalent over the Arabic words, disregarding the sense of the original." It is true that in many passages the obscurity is similar to the effect which would result if one were at this day to render idiomatic French word for word into English.

It is important to point out that the Latin of Volume I is very different from that of Vols. III-V; so different that the translation must have been the work of different persons. While the criticisms are justified with regard to these three volumes, they do not apply to the first, whose Latin is very close to the Arabic, and hardly to be improved. The difficulty really is that the Arabic itself is so condensed that the meaning can only be clearly represented in English by the use of many more words, whether to help out the meaning itself, or to make a presentable reading.

It may well be said, as did E. G. Browne, "He who judges Arabian Medicine only by the Latin translation will inevitably undervalue it and do it a great injustice. Indeed it is difficult to resist the conclusion that many passages in the Latin version of the *Qanun* of Avicenna were misunderstood or not understood at all by the translator, and consequently can never have conveyed a clear idea to the reader."[128]

The following aids to clearness have been utilized: (1) the study of Avicenna's other works, and of contemporary philosophical writings, in the existing translations. (b) The study of various Latin terms as understood by modern scholastic philosophy in its exposition of the medieval nomenclature. (c) The use of modern terms when there is no reasonable doubt of their referring to the same idea, though the literal term in the Latin is obsolete. The careful study of the original Arabic has here been of special importance, for words in the Latin version, which are evidently technical there, become merely colloquial when translated into English, whereas in the Arabic version, such words at once take on their proper character in the Arabic-English and Persian-English dictionaries (d) The use of tabulation of the matter. There are instances where this proves possible without omitting even a single Arabic word. (e) The use of paraphrase for certain passages. These are marked (p). A certain freedom of rendering has been inevitable in view of the importance of bringing the meaning of the text to the reader's notice without subjecting him to the need of reflecting deeply on passage after passage-as is requisite with the original Arabic (to have dealt with the work from the point of literature would have entailed giving the preference to safeguarding against likely criticisms at the hands of pure scholarship).

The main purpose of this treatise will now be seen to center in the idea that in the ancient philosophy there is material capable of useful application to-day. The selection of the work of Avicenna is not intended to provide an apologium for that one author, but is specially appropriate for these reasons: (i) his acknowledged excellence; (ii) his greater accessibility among medieval medical writings; (iii) a certain indefinable charm of expression peculiar to himself; but above all, (iv) the fact that his central theme is a conception of the nature of the human being really identical with that of Thomistic philosophy, and in these days specially stressed and developed by "modern scholastic philosophy." As these are related, so might Avicenna be related to a modern scholastic medicine, which would aim at reasons for health and ill health far deeper than those given by the microbic and cognate theories.

With Mercier,[129] "We do not regard the Thomistic philosophy . . . as a boundary which sets limits to personal activity of thought . . . but make use of his" (in this case, Avicenna's) "teaching as a starting-point from which we may go further afield."

With Maher,[130] we ". . . resuscitate and" (apply to medicine) ". . . a psychology that has already survived four and twenty centuries, and has had more influence on human thought and human language than all other psychologies together. My desire, however, has been not merely to expound, but to expand this old system . . . to make clear to the student of modern thought that this ancient and traditional psychology (and medicine) is not so absurd, nor these old thinkers as foolish, as current caricatures of their teaching would lead one to imagine. . . . To trespass (on the soul) . . . . is assumed by (many writers) to be the gravest of professional delinquencies."

Therefore Avicenna is allowed once more to present his theme. To the questions we are constrained to ask of him, we find our answers: (1) in his other writings; (2) in contemporary literature; (3) in the writings of modern Eastern thinkers; (4) in the works of St. Thomas; (5) in modern scholastic philosophy. If some truths are crudely expressed or perhaps faultily explained, it is our privilege to re-express and re-explain with those aids.

Those who may have failed to identify one single Truth under different garbs are not obliged to accord these garbs an unfriendly reception upon the stage of our modern world. To recall a favorite Indian metaphor, the danseuse has so robed herself, and displays such diversities of art that under the ever-changing colored beams of light it is difficult to believe there can be only one and the same artiste before us. Should it prove impossible to verify this, at least the very exhibition of the art should serve so to refresh that we can resume our work and ambitions with an added zest now confident that the future realization of our desires is not so intangible as at first appeared.

I deemed life was tranquillity and rest,
I find it but a never-ending quest;
And I, who sat in quietude and peace,
Toil on a journey that shall never cease

(Shamshad)

Why should the Cosmos turn its wheel of worlds
If not to search for Thee eternally?
Why should the tireless Sun arise each morn
If not to look for Thee?

(Zauq)

How can I win that Hidden One
Who sits within the secret place,
For even in my very dreams
She wears the veil upon Her face.

(Jurat)

For long, throughout the world, I sought for Thee,
Through weary years and ages of unrest—
At last I found Thee hidden in my arms
Within my breasts.

(Zauq)

That which is spread before us, beneath the unceasing surge and change of the crowded life of the thoroughfares of great cities, as well as beneath the panorama of nature herself, was surely understood by those who insisted " there is no second Cause," and by Chu Hsi in saying "the innumerable laws (of nature) all proceed from one source."[131] In this the thought is not pietistically of a Creator, but of a living Reality met (passively or receptively) or encountered (actively or contestingly) by us all at all times. That Reality must be understood before we handle the problem of our patient with real efficacy.

In the intention of this work, then, there comes into consideration that greater art of medicine—not an ethical Hippocratic ideal, but something of the divine—an art as real to Avicenna, philosopher, poet, musician, the worker among the great and the small, aware of the dramatic in life, as it should be to us. So we step out of the world of the modern critic, the scholar, and the medical historian, indeed of modern medicine itself, into one in which we stand, as it were, hand in hand, with the great Master of the East—almost with his very eyes gazing upon and scrutinizing this ever open book of life of ours—divested of the false notions of "progress" and "time." His language is thus no longer alien—and, incidentally, he lives again!

Avicenna's Preface

In the first place we render thanks to God, for the very excellence of the order of His creation, and the abundance of His benefits. His mercies are upon all the prophets. Secondly, is at the request of one of my special friends [was it al-Juzjani? LB], one whom I feel most bound to consider, that I prepare this book on medicine, setting forth its general and particular laws to the full extent necessary, and yet with apt brevity.

Volume I: General Medicine

My plan is to deal with the general aspects of each of the two divisions of medicine—the speculative and the practical. Then I shall treat of the general principles applicable to the diagnosis of the properties of the simples, following this with a detailed account of them. I shall, then, take up the disorders which befall each individual member, beginning with an account of its anatomy, and that of its auxiliary. The anatomy of the several members and their auxiliaries is dealt with in the first book. Having completed the account of the anatomy, I shall show how the health of the member is to be maintained.

This subject being completed, I proceed to a general discourse about general diseases: their causes, the signs by which they are recognized, and the modes of treatment. After this, I pass on to the special diseases and will point out in as many cases as possible: (1) the general diagnosis of their characters, causes and signs; (2) the special diagnostic features; (3) the general rules of treatment; (4) the special methods of treatment by (a) simples; and (b) compounded medicines.

I include specially designed tables under the subject of simples to enable you to survey the facts rapidly as to the adjuvants for treating disease by simples.

I have deemed it best to consider compounded medicines, their adjuvants, and how to mix them separately in a formulary. This it is my intention to compose after the special subjects are dealt with. Disorders not confined to one member are described in this book; cosmetics are spoken of, and the knowledge set forth in previous books is assumed. God helping me to complete this volume, the formulary will be added to it. Every follower of my teachings, who wishes to use them profitably, should memorize most of this work, even though he not understand it all.

It is my intention to prepare further volumes if God should prolong my life still further, and if circumstances prove propitious. [Avicenna was to complete five volumes of which this is the translation of the first volume. LB.]

...

A brief summary of the contents of remaining volumes, II, III, IV, and V of *The Canon* are: [Volumes I, II and V have been translated into English. LB]

Volume II: Simple Drugs

This volume gives a detailed material medical pharmacology and therapeutics of drugs. It has two parts.

Part One. General Principles: These deal with the temperament or constitution of drugs, and how it is determined: (1) by experiment; and (2) by deduction. Conditions of the experiment such as, its being on the human body, drug to be free of extrinsic and intrinsic alterations, the trial to be allopatric and made on simple diseases, drug to be qualitatively and quantitatively corresponding to the severity of the disease, etc., have been described. Part one also gives an account of all the actions which drugs may possess and describes the method of collection and preservation of the various herbal and other products.

Part Two. List of Drugs: It gives 797 drugs in seriatim according to the Abjad system. The properties of each drug have been described under the following headings: general description of the drug, tests for its purity, qualities, general and special actions on each system of the body or on special diseases; specific actions; antidotal properties; alternative remedies and adjuvants.

Volume III: Diseases of Individual Members

In Volume III, the various diseases have been discussed systematically, with their etiology, symptoms, diagnosis, prognosis and treatment with simple drugs. Special mention may be made of the following sections:

Head: brain, (intemperaments, headache in all its aspects, organic diseases of the brain, epilepsy, paralysis, etc.) eye, ear, nose, mouth, throat, and teeth. Chest: lungs, heart, breasts. Alimentary tract: stomach, intestines, liver, gall bladder and spleen. Intestines and the anus, disorders of the rectum. Urinary tract: the kidneys, bladder and urine. The male reproductive system; the female reproductive system, conception, pregnancy, and diseases of women. Muscles: joints, and feet.

Volume IV: General Diseases

Part One. Fevers: general description of fevers; their periodicity; causes such as constipation, diarrhea, dietetic indiscretion; excessive activity; excessive wakefulness; fear or anger; pain, inflammation, putrefaction, humoural disturbances; etc. Diagnosis of fevers; epidemic fevers; small pox; phthisis. Prognosis. Management of symptoms such as thirst, rigors, diarrhea, vomiting, sleeplessness, pain, headache, etc. Treatment of fevers: general and specific. Subject of crisis.

Part Two. Boils and swellings. Leprosy. Minor surgery. Wounds and their general treatment. Injuries: fractures and dislocations. Ulcers. Glandular swellings.

Part Three. Poisoning with mineral, vegetable and animal products. Bites from animals and man.

Part Four. Beauty culture. Leanness and obesity. Hair, nails and skin. Treatment of offensive odors and discolorations including leucoderma. Pediculosis. Pitting from small pox, etc.

Volume V: The Formulary

This volume gives details of special prescriptions and antidotes; their form such as pills, powders, syrups, decoctions, confections, elixirs, etc, and their method of preparation. A thorough discourse about laxatives; purgative and non-purgative powders; medicinal powders, dosages; electuaris; potions and thickened juices; jams and preserves; pills; greens and cereals; lotions; and ointments and dressings. Prescriptions for different diseases. Weights and measures.

Avicenna's Introduction
The Basis of Health and Disease and the Inevitability of Death

Medicine comprises two parts, one theoretical, and one practical, though both are really speculative science. That which is specially named theory relates to the formation of opinions and the showing of the evidence upon which they are based, without reference to the mode of acting upon them. Thus this part deals with the temperaments, the humours, the drives, and with the forms, the symptoms, and the causes of disease. That which is specially named practical relates to the mode of acting upon this knowledge, and the prescription of a regimen.

For instance, it is that part of medicine which helps us understand how the health of the body is to be maintained in this or that state, and by what means we can heal the diseases with which the body is afflicted. Practical does not refer to the performance of surgical operations. It is the art which teaches us in what way to procure healing— the healing art.

The human being takes its origin from two things: (1) the male semen, which plays the part of factor; and (2) the female menstrual discharge, which provides the matter.

Each of these is fluid and moist, but there is more wateriness and earthly substance in the female blood and female sperm, whereas air and fire are predominant in the male sperm. It is essential that at the outset of the congelation of the two components there should be moisture, even though earth and fire are found in the product. The earth provides the firmness and rigidity; the fire provides the maturative power. These give the coagulum (*"He created man from a clot"* Quran, 96:2) a certain hardness or firmness. But this hardness is not as great in degree as that possessed by a stone or glass. For these are either not soluble at all or only soluble to a degree imperceptible to our senses, however long one exposes them to solvents. Were the hardness comparable to this, the product of conception would never suffer injury however long or however persistently a solvent were applied. But that is not so. The act is contrary.

Our bodies are exposed to injury from two directions—externally and internally. The source of internal injury is the dissipation of the moisture from which we are created, and this dissipation proceeds in an orderly manner. The second source is the putrefactive breakdown and metamorphosis of the humour into a form such that the fermentative phenomena of life are no longer able to proceed.

The second source of injury differs from the first in that dryness is here introduced by virtue of depravity of humour; and this dryness continues neutralizing the moisture of the body until the form ceases to have a capacity for life.

Finally, the putrefactive breakdown disperses the vitality, because it first destroys the moisture and then disperses it, and simply dry ash is left behind.

Therefore we see that these two sources of destruction [of the living product of conception] are different from those arising from other causes —such as, freezing cold, torrid heat, grave forms of loss of continuity, various maladies. But it is in regard to the first two named sources of destruction that we find the more important factors relative to the question of the preservation of health.

Each of them takes its origin from extrinsic and intrinsic agents. The extrinsic agents are for example, the atmosphere, which is a solvent and putrefacient. The intrinsic agents are, for example, the innate heat, which is the agent within us through which moisture is dispersed: the extraneous heat generated within us from the aliments, and through other agents which cause putrefactive changes in the [native] moistures.

All these agents mutually aid one another in rendering the body dry. And yet it is true that our perfection and soundness and the power to perform our various actions depend on a degree of dryness of the blood. But the degree of dryness becomes relatively greater and greater until we die. Therefore, this dryness is inevitable.

If we were at the outset essentially composed of moisture, heat would have to overcome it or else the heat would be choked by it. Therefore the heat continues to exert its own effect, that is, it produces more and more desiccation. But whatever degree of dryness there might be at the outset (of life), it reaches equilibrium, and remains so until the limit of equilibrium in regard to dryness is reached. The heat remaining constant, the dryness is now relatively greater than before for the matter is less, and hence holds more.

Therefore it is not difficult to understand that the dryness passes on beyond the stage of equilibrium, and goes on steadily increasing until the whole of the moisture of the body is consumed. Therefore (we may say) that the innate heat is the cause of its own extinction, for it is itself the reason for its own matter being consumed. We may compare it to the flame of a lamp; the light goes out when all the matter has been used up.

As the dryness increases, the innate heat diminishes. The loss continues unceasingly till death, and the moisture which is lost is not restored. The loss goes on more and more.

The dryness (of the body) is increased in two ways: by lessening of the power of receiving matter; by lessening of the native moisture resulting from dispersal of the (innate) heat. The heat becomes more feeble because dryness predominates in the substance of the members, and because the innate moisture becomes relatively less. The innate moisture is to the innate heat as the oil of a lamp is to the flame. For there are two forms of moisture in the flame: water, which holds its own, and oil, which is used up. So, in a corresponding manner, the innate heat holds its own in respect of the innate moisture, but is used up *pari passu* with increase of extraneous heat, due, for example, to defective digestion, which is comparable with the aqueous moisture of the flame. As the dryness increases, the innate heat lessens, and the result is natural death.

For the reason why the (human) body does not live any longer than it does lies in the fact that the initial innate moisture holds out against being dispersed both by the alien heat and by the heat in the body itself (both that which is innate and that derived from bodily movement). And this resistance is maintained as long as the one is weaker than the other, and as long as something is provided to replace that which has been thus dispersed, to wit, from the aliment. Furthermore, as we have already stated, the power or drive which operates upon the aliment in order to render it useful in this way only does so up to the end of life.

Therefore, we may say that the art of maintaining health is not the art of averting death or of averting extraneous injuries from the body or of securing the utmost longevity possible to the human being. It is concerned with two other things: (1) the prevention of putrefactive breakdown; and (2) the safeguarding of innate moisture from too rapid dissipation and maintaining it at such a degree of strength that the original type of constitution peculiar to the person shall not change even up to the last moment of life.

This is secured by a suitable regimen, namely: (a) one which will ensure the replacement of the innate heat and moisture which are dispersed from the body as exactly as possible; and (b) a regimen which will prevent any agents which would lead to a rapid dessication from gaining the upper hand excluding agents which produce a normal desiccation; (c) one which safeguards the body from the development of putrefactive processes within it and from the influence of alien heat (whether extraneous or intrinsic) because all bodies have not the same degree of innate moisture and innate heat. There is a great diversity in regard to them.

Moreover, every person has his own term of life, during which the desiccation inevitable to his temperament (constitution) and the degree of innate heat, and of innate moisture can be withstood.

Nevertheless, factors may arise which assist desiccation, or are injurious in some other way. For which reason, many assert that the former are natural causes of death, whereas the latter are accidental. And under this view, the art of maintaining health consists in guiding the body to its natural span of life by paying attention to whatever things conduce thereto. There are two drives to be fostered by the doctor in striving for this object: (1) the nutritive drive whereby that is replaced which is constantly being lost to the body namely earthiness and aquosity; and (2) the sensitive drive (animal faculty), that is, the pulsatile faculty which is concerned with the replacement of that which is lost to the body by the breath namely air and fire. And since aliments are only potentially like the thing nourished, an alternative drive had to be created so that they could be changed actually into the likeness of the thing nourished. In this way the aliment becomes effective.

The instruments and channels necessary for this had to be created also—namely the means by which material is attracted, expelled, retained, and digested (sequence by sequence, turn by turn).

Therefore, we may say that the essential considerations in the art of preserving the health consist in maintaining equilibrium between all these various concomitant factors. But there are seven matters concerning which special care must be expended to ensure just proportion: (1) equilibrium of temperament; (2) selection of the articles of food and drink; (3) evacuation of effete matters; (4) safeguarding the composite; (5) maintaining the purity of the air respired; (6) guarding against extraneous contingencies; and (7) moderation in regard to the movements of the body and the motions of the mind, with which may be included sleep and wakefulness.

From all these considerations you will now perceive that there is no single fixed limit to which equilibrium or health is to be assigned. None of the temperaments enters into it. Health and equilibrium vary (in range) from time to time. That is to say, it is a state comprised—within two limits.

On the Breath

1.1. General Remarks

God created the left side of the heart and made it hollow in order that it should serve both as a storehouse of the breath and as the seat of manufacture of the breath. He also created the breath to enable the drives of the "soul' to be conveyed into the corresponding members. In the first place the breath was to be the rallying-point for the faculties of the soul and in the second place it was to be an emanation into the various members and tissues of the body (whereby these could manifest the functions of those drives).

Now He produced the breath out of the finer particles of the humours and out of heat and dryness (fire) and at the same time produced the tissues themselves (the visible body) out of the coarser and cold and dry (earthy) particles of these humours. In other words, the breath is related to the attenuated particles as the body is related to the coarser particles of the same humours. Just as the humours are intermingled to produce a temperamental "form," whereby the members of the body are enabled to receive a physical appearance, impossible were they separate, so the attenuated portions of the humours, being intermingled into a temperamental form, enable the breath to receive the powers of the soul —impossible were the humours separate.

The beginning of the breath is as a divine emanation from potentiality to actuality proceeding without intermission or stint until the form (preparation, state) is completed and perfected. Each member, though derived from the self-same substance of the humours, nevertheless has its own particular temperament—for the proportional qualities of the (denser portions of the) humours and the form of their commixture are peculiar to each member. Similarly, although derived from the same attenuated portions of the humours, nevertheless each of the three breaths (natural, animal and vital) has its own particular temperament, because the proportional quantities of the more attenuated portions of the humours and the manner of their commixture are peculiar to each breath.

Although the body consists of several organs, there is one from which they all originally arose. As to what this organ actually was, there are various opinions. The fact remains that one organ necessarily came to light before other organs could arise out of it. Exactly the same is true in the case of the breaths. There is one single breath which accounts for the origin of the others. This breath, according to the most important philosophers, arises in the heart, passes thence into the principal centers of the body, lingering in them long enough to enable them to impart to it their respective temperamental properties. Lingering in the cerebrum it receives a temperament whereby it is capable of receiving the drives of sensation and movement; in the liver, it receives the drive of nutrition and growth (vegetative drives); in the generative glands it acquires a temperament which prepares it for receiving the drive of generation (reproduction).

The foundation or beginning of all these drives is traceable to the heart as is agreed upon even by those philosophers who think that the source of visual, auditory and gustatory power lies in the brain.

Some philosophers consider that the breath is made able to receive these drives and so be perfected in other organs than those named. Thus, visual power results from the union of the temperament of the breath with the moist temperament of the crystalline lens, that the auditory power results from the union thereof with the temperament of the auditory nerve; that gustatory power is produced by the mediation of the moist temperament afforded by the soft spongy sub-lingual glands.

Others reject this view and consider that the earth carries the faculty or drives from the brain and receives nothing from the temperament of the member to which it travels, as nothing is necessary to perfect it. The member itself is an instrument well adapted for the action of the vegetative drive and contributes nothing of its own essence.

1.2. The Nature of the Breath and Its Purpose

Life and every perfection and every goods for which creatures are destined, comes from nothing but the primal Truth—the source of all good and from the strong desire ever proceeding therefrom

Nevertheless, the recipient thereof requires a specific capacity for reception of the good. A creature cannot receive indifferently. For instance, wool cannot be wool (lit., half the "form" of wool) and at the same time have the character of a sword. Water cannot be water (lit., have the "form" of water) and at the same time receive the "form" of human nature.

All corporeal bodies may receive life, except the four first principles, and whatever is of like nature to them. For these are non-living bodies, and are also of negligible bulk. In fact their bulk is infinitesimal compared with the planets, and still more strikingly so compared with some of the fixed stars. Indeed it can be shown that these first principles in their totality have not as much bulk as a point compared with the body of Saturn; how mulch less then are they when compared with the higher bodies?

Those who realize the Truth know the reason why these elementary bodies do not receive the "form" of life. Even the simplest of living beings is quite different from them; and the celestial bodies, adapted as they are to a very wonderful kind of corporeal life, are very different from them also. The first-principles are entirely beyond the possibility of life.[1]

It is the mingling of substances in the compound bodies which accounts for their ability to receive life. The commingling of the components so modifies their contrarieties as to produce an ensemble (i.e., the temperament), in which all the various seeming contraries [nothing is really absolutely contrary to anything else—a typical Sufi concept] are blended harmoniously. The more harmonious the blending, the more adapted is the resultant compound for being the vehicle, not merely of life, but of a very particular kind of life. Perfect equilibrium and perfect balance renders possible the manifestation of the perfection of rational life which celestial beings possess. And it is just this kind of character which is to be found in the case of the human breath!

The breath, then, is that which emerges from a mixture of first principles, and approaches towards the likeness of celestial beings. It is a luminous substance. It is a ray of light.

This accounts for the fact that the mind rejoices when it looks towards the light, and is depressed when exposed to darkness. Light is in harmony with the breath. Darkness is in discord with it.

1.3. The Common Emotions in Relation to the Vital Breath:
Their First Causes: Potentiality and Disposition

Sages and those physicians who agree with them, are satisfied that joy and sadness, fear and anger, are passions peculiarly; related to the breath of the heart. Each of these emotions is maintained or discontinued: (1) by the agent [in the scholastic sense]; (2) by the persistence or cessation of the disposition exhibited by the substance of the patient.

Sages perceive a subtle distinction between potentiality and disposition.[2]

1.3.1. Joy and the Causes of Delight and Sadness

Joy is a form of delight. A thing is delightful when it is the perfection of its corresponding faculty or drive. For instance, the perception of a sweet or sapid taste or a pleasant fragrance; the overruling of a feeling of anger by a good judgment; the realization of some useful outcome of the reasoning or imaginative drive.

There is a certain power accruing from every perfected delight. It is the perfection of the given power which produces joy.[3]

Some people have expressed the opinion that delight is really nothing but the departure of abnormal disposition, and that there cannot possibly be delight where there is no possibility of going beyond the natural disposition. This view has arisen because there are some forms of power which cannot bring delight until some abnormal disposition has first been eliminated. Nevertheless this opinion is wrong; it takes a thing which is an accident for a thing per se—a fallacy of reasoning which is mentioned in "the definitions."

Delight[4] implies attaining a goal, and the one who apprehends it can only be aware of the delight because he is aware of the change. For instance: (1) in the case of touch, it is evident that the quality of tangibility can only provide delight as long as the tactile organ continues to be in the opposite phase. Once the polarity has reached equilibrium, the character of the organ will have become "setup" and cannot provide further change. From this time there ceases to be any sensation of pleasure. (2) In the case of the hectic patient who does not suffer from heat subjectively however high the body temperature may be, a patient with an acute fever may feel hotter than the other even though his temperature be not so high. This is because in the hectic case, heat is already resident in tissues of the corresponding constitution; in acute fevers, it is as if the heat flew past, afraid of the manner in which it may find the elements mingled in the tissues. Doctors rightly consider the state of the members of a hectic case as "bad, though balanced," and in the other case regard the quality as "unbalanced and therefore bad."

It is clear then that pleasure ceases as soon as one is accustomed to the completed sense perception because one can now no longer be aware of the entry of sense perceptions. The reason why pleasure is experienced at the departure of an abnormal disposition is that one is now sensitive to the slightest change in the now normal disposition. It is possible that this sensitiveness to change in the natural disposition may appear synchronously with the departure of the abnormal disposition. People are then apt to think the latter was the cause of the former when it is not so. The real explanation lies in the attainment of perfect perception. It is this that is the intrinsic basis of delight.[5]

In other words, the disposition towards delight depends on the constitution of the participating breaths, and on the degree to which the disposition is favorable to their presence always provided that the substance of the breath is not diminished, and the disposition likely to be favorable is not an abnormal one.

The effect of quantity of breath—should a breath with a tendency towards delight be abundant, its action will be correspondingly powerful, the greater its vigor, and the greater is the amount of it which will persist at the place of its origin—that is, in its "matrix." Consequently, under these circumstances it will radiate out in greater measure to the various members and produce that particular state of expansion which spells joy and pleasure. For, if the breath in question were only moderate in amount, the substrate concerned would hold it greedily, and not allow it to expand as freely as otherwise would be the case.

The effect of the quality of the breath—the more noble the character possessed by it and the more noble its substance, the more luminous does it become, and the more like celestial substance will it be.[6]

Such, then, are the various points about the tendency towards pleasure and joy. As regards sorrow and grief, it is just a question of the converse. Once the general sources of delight and pleasure are thoroughly grasped, the sources of joy become intelligible, since joy is a form of delight.

By way of summary, it may be said that when the breath residing in the heart is plentiful (as it is when there is plenty of that material from which it is rapidly and constantly being generated); when it is balanced in temperament; when it has a luminous, beautiful and bright substance then there is a strong tendency to joy.

When the breath is scanty (as occurs in convalescents, in long-standing illnesses, and in elderly persons); when it is not balanced in character (as in morbid states); and when it is: (a) very dense and coarse in substance (as in melancholy and elderly people), it cannot arouse joy; (b) very delicate in substance (as in convalescents and in women), it will not allow of expansion; and (c) confused (as in melancholy people). In all these cases there is a very strong tendency to depression, sadness and grief.[7]

1.3.2. The External Causes of Delight and Sadness

When all the conditions required for a given act are present, the slightest agent will now suffice to effect the act. Thus, when sulphur is used for kindling, it is because sulphur is set afire by a moderate amount of heat, whereas wood cannot be made to burn without twice as much. So, when the mind has a breath whose tendency to receive the impress of gladdening agents is complete, a slight agent will suffice to evoke gladness.

The action of wine on emotions and on breath—this is shown in the instance of those who drink excellent wine, for in such persons gladness increases to such a pitch that onlookers wonder how they can be jovial without reason. Such a thing, of course, cannot be. No impression is possible without an impresser.

But the fact is that when wine is taken in moderation, it gives rise to a large amount of breath, whose character is balanced, and whose luminosity is strong and brilliant. Hence wine disposes greatly to gladness, and the person is subject to quite trivial exciting agents. The breath now takes up the impression of agents belonging to the present time more easily than it does those which relate to the future; it responds to agents conducive to delight rather than those conducive to a sense of beauty. It also takes up an impression from agents which are prone to evoke conjecture rather than from those which are concerned with real understanding. The explanation of this is that normally the power of the mind brings about an act in the brain such as will expel the breath (when it is in the phase of having a mild degree of moisture); the brain thus becomes able to obey the motions of the thought and the exercise of the faculty of understanding. In inebriety, however, there is a very great inclination towards excess of moisture (which is incompatible with obedience to the understanding), owing to admixture with ascending and overflowing vapors, which render it too humid. This moisture prevents it from obeying the intellectual faculty and the tendencies of the thought, except in respect of very material and corporeal topics. It cannot serve in respect of very delicate spiritual matters. Whether stable or agitated, moisture cannot take part in the formation or presentation of spiritual affairs; it can only respond to corporeal ones.

The stages in inebriety: the following are the various steps of degradation of the mind, not arranged chronologically: First, recognition of truth is impaired, and the operation of the mind is imperfect. The intellectual power falls in proportion. The substrate continues to attract breath until the temperament of one has reached up to that of the other after which the flow of breath of course comes to an end.

The power of the mind—which is in the "heart"— has a greater affinity for joy during the state of drunkenness; the gladdening things that come to it do not reach it by the usual route between the senses and fantasy (or even the cogitative faculty or drive), because the sensitive drives have come into dominance. The repletion of the breath with moisture has altered its vigor. The senses now dominate the inner breath, and are more powerful than the understanding. The understanding (as, for instance, for geometry and other exact sciences), meeting as it does a breath which is so wanton towards it, unreadily submits to the senses. Things being so, no wonder that the conception of future, of beauty, of rational affairs, has become blurred in the intoxicated person's mind; the sense perception of sweet, glad, and delectable things prevails, and the sense of the present is very strong. It is the very strength of this tendency that accounts for the fact that quite a slight agent will evoke gladness and mirth. Onlookers think that such persons are jovial without reason. But this cannot be so. As a matter of fact, some causative agents of joy and gladness are powerful, while others are weak; some are known and obvious, others are not known and occult. Many of the latter are not known, not because they occur only rarely do they occur regularly. The fact is that we notice things less particularly the more often we encounter them.

It is now necessary to detail the powerful and obvious sources of joy and gladness. Instances of sources of joy are the following: (1) gazing upon the daylight, among cheerful people. The evidence of this is that being in the dark makes them sad; (2) having intercourse with those of like beliefs. The evidence of this is that solitude makes such people sad. Gladdening influences are things such as: (3) obtaining that which is wished for; (4) satisfying an intention without meeting opposition; (5) preferring to do something peaceful, (6) confidence; (7) the memory of past and future joys and hopes; (8) thinking about ambitious things; (9) mutual argumentation with kindred minds; (10) relief from pain; (11) contact with curious (interesting, unusual, remarkable, new) things; (12) uplifting of the mind; (13) meeting friends and friendly surroundings; (14) overcoming deception in small matters; and many similar things to be found mentioned in books of rhetoric and morals.[8]

All these vary in different races according to their affections, habits and ages. None of them is invariably absent. If two agents usually having a gladdening effect occur together the effect is not so much the greater. All that happens is that the disposition is more drawn to one than the other. The effect of one only overrules that of the other if the agent in question be very powerful, or, if it be weak, only if it be very persistently at work. This accounts for delight being able to persist during the state of inebriation, and for the fact that melancholy persons with confused breaths keep sad after agencies producing a sense of desolation and sadness—such as the following: (1) reflecting that one's homeland is distant; (2) pondering over many injuries already past and done with; (3) hate and rancor; (4) bad health; (5) difficult circumstances of life; (6) thinking terrible things are going to happen in the future; (7) thinking of the necessity for death, which natural judgment ignores because of the obvious fact-—that we must die; (8) thinking about something that it is disturbing to meditate upon; (9) being away from an agreeable occupation; (10) having thoughts that distract from one's occupation; (11) distraction from that which is desired for and wished for; (12) many other similar things, and others which are beyond comprehension. Things of this sort easily sadden a mind which is disposed to become sad. Moreover, in melancholy persons the vividness of the imagination of depressing things itself causes (them to appear, because the thing whose image is represented to the mind is already there in actuality. Hence depression persists.

Vividness of imagination goes with dryness of the breath, the movement of which the will has power to correct. We find that the understanding is drawn away from rational actions by the senses and by the fantasies whenever the character of the breath is perverted; for the breath moves characteristically towards that direction in which a lack of congenial disposition arises, as when the quality of the breath is very bad, and when it is confused.

1.3.3. How Each Emotion Tends to Generate its Own Type of Breath

It is not to be thought that every agent tending towards joy or depression necessarily depends only on the quantity or quality of the substance of the breath. Other agencies are concerned. For instance, the emotions of the mind have to be considered. These tend to one or other of the aforesaid, true though it be that they act through the agency of factors internal in the breath itself (namely, quantity, quality) They do this by modifying the temperamental substrate or by rectifying the breath or by increasing its quantity Thus, they dispose towards joy. On the other hand, an agent of the opposite sign will tend to induce depression. These are the immediate and remote, external factors.

The internal factors are traceable to one single source, because every act of contrary type, if it be repeated often, comes to be more efficient in imparting an effect Every increment of power carries with it so much more tendency to the accomplishment of the effect. This is sufficiently plain from a purely logical point of view. A body which is very heating tends to impart heat rapidly; and similarly—in the case of cold, rare and dense bodies. The same holds good in the case of the internal potencies. This is how it is that a strong character is formed by repeated practice and repeated experience of emotion. It is in this way that moral character is acquired. Perhaps the reason underlying this is that when an emotion appears, it often makes the substance of the breath become conducive; and what is suitable for one thing is unsuitable for its opposite. The more often it is repeated, the less does the tendency to the opposite become, for that which is conducive to the opposite, is expelled little by little. This is saying the same thing as logic says. It would be tedious to prove it by syllogism by an acceptable and convincing argument from known premises. It emerges from the aforesaid that a reiteration of being glad disposes the breath to a state of gladness; a reiteration of being sad disposes it to depression.

Natural enquiry shows the source of increase of gladness to depend on: (1) a strengthening of the natural faculty: (2) a rarefaction of the breath—the latter is due to the expansion following gladness: (2) the strengthening of the natural drive is contributed to by three factors, each of which is itself a source of gladness; (a) the temperament of the breath; (b) overproduction of the breath beyond that which is lost by dispersal; (c) prevention of excessive dispersal of breath. Rarefaction of the breath is followed by two things: (i) a tendency towards movement and expansion—this is related to the fineness (rarefaction) of its substance; and (ii) an attraction to itself of its own particular nutriment.

This is due to the movement of expansion towards a place away from the movement of the nutriment. This particular attraction is really the natural corporeal tendency to avoid emptiness. In its essence, it is the same with any movement which in itself brings it to pass that the latter things shall take the place of the former. It is the outcome of this law that very distant waters are drawn towards their primary source, and that winds follow the course they do.

Two things follow great depression: (1) weakening of natural power; and (2) concentration of the breath. The explanation of this is that violent condensation and aggregation of the breath obliterates the natural heat and results in coldness. Two opposites follow upon this, as has already been intimated.

It is therefore evident that intense gladness disposes the breath to gladness, sadness to depression; that associated depressants do not make an impression on gladness unless they are vigorous; whereas weak stimulants may and do impress themselves thereon. It is, of course, the other way about in the case of depressants.

1.3.4. The Distinction Between Weakness of the Heart and Cowardice, Sadness and Their Opposites

Weakness of the heart and sadness, which some people call "contraction of the chest or heart," are similar and yet different. The same thing may be said about their opposites (vigor and gladness of heart), which some people call "enlargement of the chest or heart.[9] The difference between them is difficult to identify because so commonly one passes into the other. Most people think the two former are passive dispositions; others think they are active. But there is an obvious difference between the extremes of each: (1) Not every weak heart is associated with depression nor is depression always accompanied by a weak heart. A vigorous heart is not necessarily accompanied by joy; and conversely. (2) The basis is different in each. Weakness of the heart is a disposition assumed in respect of things evoking dread, because it is incapable of tolerating them. Depression has to do with saddening things and the heart does not tolerate them much. Fear concerns the body; depression concerns the mind. (3) There is a difference in regard to the mental effect. Weakness of the heart impels to flight; depression impels one to stand still for the purpose of either resisting or repelling. This is the opposite action to flight. Weakness of the heart inhibits the powers of motion; depression stimulates them. Consequently there are two emotions associated with weakness of the heart: (a) that of a threatening injury; and (b) that of the desire to prolong movement. In the case of depression (oppression of the chest) there are: (i) a sense of threatening injury; (ii) no desire to flee. In the event of there being a decision to flee, it is because of some contingent circumstance rather than because of an intention to give ground. It is as likely that attack and struggle will be decided upon in place of flight. (4) They differ as to the after effects on the body. Weakness of the heart and escape from danger are followed by loss of natural heat, by cold. Depression, after the particular cause has passed away, is followed by kindling of the natural heat. (5) They differ in regard to the disposing causes. Too fine and too cold a complexioned breath tends to weakness of the heart; coarseness and hot temperament of the breath tend to depression.[10]

1.3.5. The Relations Between the Various Blood States and the Several Emotions

The part played by imagination in emotions—the persistence of an imagination which s disposed towards taking vengeance for a thing is related to persistence of anger although there is not sufficient propulsive power to execute the vengeance. The anger is neither marked enough nor mild enough. For it must be understood that when anger ceases quickly, the hurtful image does not persist in the imagination, but is quickly destroyed; so rancor becomes impossible.

In like manner, too much tendency to secure vengeance is countered by two factors: rancor and hate. The one is due to the mind being wholly impelled to vengeance, but prevented from continually reflecting upon the hurtful conditions by remembering the things which follow upon having hate fixed in the memory. The mind naturally hesitates to face impending hurts. Externals tend to draw away from internals and vice versa.

It must also be remembered that when there is too much tendency to vengeance in a fearless person, the impression results as if the imagination had already become possessed of the thing desired for. In aiming at the realization of a power, and hastening towards it, the imagination of such a person takes it as actually handled. The image is impressed on the imagination as if actually present; then the image of the thing in which the purposed action will end is added to the imagination, and the desire for it ceases to be maintained; the image is abolished, and therefore does not linger in the memory. That is how it is that rancor is not there.

When the noxa is big, as where a sultan or very high dignitary (usually looked on with fear) is concerned, then the urgent anxiety to gain vengeance, coupled with the fear, together prevent the image of the desire from staying in the mind. The result is that the picture of the desire and of the noxa are both abolished from the imagination, whereas the image of the fear is so much the more dominant to the mind that it evokes a desire to flee and not attack. Here again, the image of rancor cannot persist in the mind. In the case of persons under puberty, or weakly persons, it is so easy to take vengeance on them, and there is so little fear entertained of them that the vengeful mind pictures the vengeance as if already accomplished. Excessive ease in securing vengeance makes it pictured as if already in one's hand. The imagination acts not according to what is in the matter at issue, but according to that which it pictures to itself. So, when ease of fulfillment arouses the thought that vengeance is attained, the weak-minded person takes it as actually attained. So the love for it vanishes and is entirely obliterated from the mind.

Moreover, that the imagination moves according to that which is represented to it and not according to the outcome of things, is shown by the fact that men dislike honey when it is served up like bilious matter; and they dislike laudable sapid foods should their color be made like repugnant substances: or even when they are served in the appearance of repugnant objects even though such things are not believed to exist at all.

Similarly with this: when a given likeness to the above named thing is portrayed (either because of the intensity of the impulse of the desire, or because of the worthlessness of realizing the desire as though it had actually been attained) it has the same effect as if it had been realized; therefore there is no rancor.

From what has been said in the preceding chapter, it is evident that the last-named kind of temperament is that which is most disposed towards rancor.

1.3.6. How the Appropriate Medicines Stimulate And Strengthen the Breath

We can now understand how the appropriate medicines can stimulate. Wine, for instance, restores the breath by nourishing it; pearl and silk (which counteracts disagreeable things) supply the breath with brilliance and luminosity. Embolic myrobalan, amber, and coral concentrate the breath or prevent it from dissipating rapidly; doronicum modifies the temperament of the breath by giving it heat; camphor and rose-water do so by imparting cold; sweet aromatics strengthen the breath by endowing its substance with agreeable and sweet fragrance; bugloss and lapis lazuli act by separating off black bile and fumosity. Changes are produced by adding or removing a drug; i.e., coral may be joined with amber and bugloss.

In some cases, gladness is the outcome of the intrinsic property of the drug. This is so in the case of sunbul. In other cases, the intrinsic property of the drug produces its effect indirectly by acting upon one or other of the primary causes of gladness. Thus, musk and amber act on the breath by way of their aromaticity. The juice of matian gives rise to gladness by virtue of an intrinsic property. But when used in a case where the temperament of the breath is hot, the stimulant action is effected by way of infrigidation. When the temperament of the breath is cold, doronicum acts as stimulant both by virtue of its intrinsic property and by imparting warmth to the breath.

In dealing with all these drugs, then, it is necessary to know whether the properties are general or specific. When the property is general there is no need to make any modifications in employing it for weakness or depression of the heart. An instance of such an agent is afforded by aromaticity. On the other hand, where the property is specific, it requires modification. For instance, the juice or syrup of matianus is cold, and will stimulate one kind of temperament but not another. If it be desired to use matianus to make a person of cold temperament glad, it is necessary to counteract its coldness by a calefacient; and it would be more efficient to choose a calefacient which itself is intrinsically a stimulant. For instance, musk or amber is mixed with syrup of matian, because they supply both warmth and stimulating power.

Aromaticity and sweetness are potencies which, though opposite, are yet attracted towards qualities which are agreeable to the substance of the breath. They supply the taste and fragrance which the natural and vital power respectively desire to receive.

Where two drugs are of equal power, the sweeter and more aromatic of the two will prove a more efficient adjuvant, because these properties are more attractive to the members (especially the liver). Should nutrient properties be present as well, the breath is more rapidly nourished; and being medicinal in character, it acts more rapidly on the breath.

These indications guide as to which drugs to use to obtain a more rapid effects.

The essence of aromaticity lies in its rarefaction; the essence of sweetness lies in its concentration and earthiness. This explains why aromatics are so much better adapted to feed the breath, while sweet substances are better fitted to nourish the body. Consequently aromaticity is more efficient for the heart than sweetness, while it is the other way round in the case of the liver. The heart is the matrix of generation of the nutriment of the breaths, whereas the liver is the matrix of generation of the nutriment of the body. That is why it needs less aromaticity and more sweetness to nourish it than does the heart. All the same, aromaticity is required by the liver, because that organ is the matrix of the natural breath—not a matrix of generation of the breath, only a substrate for the breath to reside in (according to those acquainted with the truth; not according to those who merely speculate).

The natural breath has a desire for aromaticity and is invigorated and refreshed by such. It is easy to-see that the natural faculties will also be invigorated in consequence.

1.3.7. What "Property" Means and How It Differs from "Nature"

Strictly speaking, the specific "property" of a thing is the same as its "nature." The one term would really be defined by the same word as the other. The specific property is the source of movement or rest in whatever thing it occurs.

Nevertheless, there is a difference between the two concepts in the same way as the particular differs from the universal. It is not true, as the laity think, that the two terms belong to opposite things. The truth is that the first principles behind all generable and corruptible substances are primary, active or kinetic energies and occur either simply in fire, air, water, and earth, or linked to a composite temperament.

There are two views about this: (1) that the disposition appears synchronously with the production of physical form; (2) that the disposition is inherent in matter from the outset. Once matter assumes a given physical form, it can only assume some other form by dispersing the first form. That is, matter relapses to the natural power of the disposition.

Whichever view is correct, it is true that from such a physical form (whose constituents have become so to say blended) there emerges a power which could not have appeared in the several separate constituents. For instance, the attractive power of iron in a magnet is not in any of its component powers. It arises out of the divine emanation which pervades all things and makes latent energies kinetic. This happens in one of two ways: (1) by means of something primarily inherent in matter; or (2) by means of the temperament which itself disposes it to receive the given power, and is yet itself neither power nor physical form.

We now have the answer to the questions, what is "specific property?" What is "nature?" If one asks, "Why does fire burn?," one must needs answer, "because the thing burning has a combustible nature." If one asks, "Why does a magnet attract iron?," it can only be said, "It has an attractive power by nature." To say that fire burns because of heat is no better than saying a magnet attracts iron because of having the power and nature to attract iron; we may say the nature of the energy called "heat" is to burn up in fire, and call this "combustible nature," "combustible power," but there is no name for the other. The giving of a name has not imparted complete know- ledge about the matter; to know the name does not remove the real lack of knowledge about a difficult phenomenon.

But people are not usually satisfied by the preceding answer because they want to believe that every property arises out of the "heat," "cold," "dryness," or "moisture" of a body by virtue of heaviness or lightness or movement or of any of the things which are obviously really dependent upon the components. When they find that actions are not to be attributed to any of the aforesaid, and that the real reason for an act is not apparent, they come to the conclusion that every one of the first beginnings is inscrutable. That is not true. Actions proceed either from natural, vital, intellectual or accidental (contingent) properties.

We may pass over as untrue the other theories held about magnetic force that it attracts iron because of: (1) heat; (2) cold; (3) a spirit residing in the magnet itself; (4) sending out hook-shaped bodies; (5) likeness between the nature of the magnet and the nature of the iron; or (6) a vacuum in the iron. The fallacy in all these ideas is easily seen when we reflect on how a green twig acquires nutritive properties from its constitution, which is the same sort of thing as the reception of magnetic properties from a constitution in the iron. What is not understood is why the magnetic power is so much greater in iron than in any other thing; yet this ignorance is no greater than that which exists in reference to other matters.

This ignorance is in two directions: (1) we do not know the initial factors which go to produce this attractive power. Neither do we know them in regard to any other force; (2) we do not know why this body is more disposed to take on magnetic power than any other body. But neither do we know more in regard to other phenomena. We are in exactly the same case concerning colors, fragrance, powers of the mind, and such like matters. Of course we can say that all such phenomena arise out of the active principles originally blessed by God, and we can allow that the basis of the disposition which comes from the particular constitution is due to a rearrangement of matter. But though we may guess that it is the proportions of ingredients which account for the existence of a temperament, it is quite another thing to be definite about the absolute proportions of this commixture, and we shall be ignorant of this as long as we live in this world. So it is evident that our ignorance of the real causes of the power in the magnet is not as remarkable as our ignorance of the real causes which dispose the corporeal or mental body to redness or yellowness.

The fact is that we take little interest in the common things of life; the mind neglects to study them; so often is it true that the rare things are the ones to excite admiration and be inquired after and their causes speculated about.

In conclusion, "specific property" is the "nature" met with in compound substances after a characteristic temperament (and its correspondingly special and characteristic state) has been initiated in them out of the supreme and limitless influence. This is the real truth about specific property. In spite of this being so, it is common for people to say that specific property differs from "nature" in that the former appears in complex bodies after a special act has occurred to make its nature manifest. On the other hand, the "nature" of a thing is said to be the power by which simple bodies are operated. This is as far as the laity and feeble searchers-after-truth can see. If fire is a difficult thing to make, and is carried from distant places, surely the laity might wonder at the specific properties of this more than of other things, and look more closely into the causes of its specific property than they do into those of other phenomena that appear to be more remarkable. To think how fire removes visible forms, cannot be touched, rises upward, makes the things over which it can prevail, ascend, can be generated from a small quantity in large amounts within an hour, destroys whatever it meets and transmutes it into its own essence, is not lessened by however much is taken from it. Surely these facts are more wonderful than the attraction of iron by a magnet, or than other specific properties. But, being so common, seen so much everyday, these things evoke no admiration. There is no interest displayed in seeking their explanation. The action of the magnet seems extraordinary and receives universal wonder, and everyone is interested in inquiring into its nature and origin.

Endnotes
Introduction by Laleh Bakhtiar

1 Seyyed Hossein Nasr, *Three Muslim Sages*, pp. 23-24.
2 The Islamic medical tradition is the part of reference of this great textbook of Avicenna (Ibn Sina) which served to heal millions of people as this was the only medical textbook for 700 years in Europe alone. Translated into Latin, it served as the basis for Shakespere's psychology, among others. St. Thomas Aquinas has said: Anything Avicenna says is correct.
3 Nader Ardalan and Laleh Bakhtiar, *The Sense of Unity*, p. 11.
4 Ibid., p. 11.
5 Ibid., p. 13.
6 Ibid.,p. 13.
7 Ibid., p. 19.
8. R. A. Nicholson, *Rumi, Mystic and Poet*, p. 31.
9. Nader Ardalan and Laleh Bakhtiar, *op. cit.*, p. 19.
10 *Ibid.*, p. 19 which quotes S. H. Nasr, *Three Muslim Sages*, p. 112.
11 Seyyed Hossein Nasr, *Islamic Science: An Illustrated Study*, p. 161.
12 According to the Ayurvedic system, there are three bio-energies called *dosha (arkan)*. They are *vatha* [nervous spirit]: driving force. It relates mainly to the nervous system and the body's energy; *pitta* [animal spirit, fire] relates to digestion, metabolism, enzymes, acid and bile; *kapha* [natural spirit] relates to mucous membranes, phlegm, moisture, fat and lymphatics.

Seyyed Hossein Nasr points out: "It is worth drawing attention to the similarity between the words *ruh* and *rih* (the wind or air) in Arabic and to the Galenic doctrine that through the air breathed by the organism the life-force enters the body. It is also of significance to note that in Arabic as in many other languages the words for breath (*nafas*) and soul (*nafs*) are related. Therein lies a profound cosmological principle which is also related to the invocation of the Name of God (*dhikr*) as the central technique of Sufism for spiritual realization." *Sufi Essays*, p.27.
13 Seyyed Hossein Nasr, *Science and Civilization in Islam*, pp. 223-224.
14 Called *prana* or energy of life in the Ayurvedic system, it is comprised of energy which changes according to our circumstances, our diet, our lifestyles and the world around us. Some are positive and some are negative. We have to live in a way to attain energy balance. Energy controls the functions of every cell, thought, emotion, and action.

O.Cameron Gruner's Remarks

1 This was actually Gruner's conclusion, but because it explains the content of The Canon so well and because today we have grown so distant from Avicenna's concepts, we have placed it before Gruner's original introduction, which follows and expounds the differences between Avicenna and "modern medicine."
2 Altounyan, Lancet, I928, ii, 684.
3 St. Thomas Aquinas, *Summa Theologica*, p. 177.
4 See Introduction by O. Cameron Gruner, Doctrine of "the Constitution"
5 See notes to Avicenna *on Psychology*, Details Regarding the Emotions.
6 See Avicenna *on Diagnosis Signs and Symptoms*, Details Regarding Odor.
7 See Avicenna *on The Temperaments*, Details Regarding Age.
8 Notes to Avicenna *On the Four Temperamen*ts, Application of the Doctrine; notes to Avicenna *on Psychology*, Details Concerning Some of the Drives; List of Terms Applicable to Mental Faculties.
9 Notes to *On His Psychology*, List of Terms Applicable to Mental Faculties.
10 St. Thomas Aquinas, *Summa Theologica*, p. 203.
11 See Avicenna *on the Breath*.
12 For other cycles see Avicenna *on Illness*.
13 See Introduction by O. Cameron Gruner, Doctrine of "the Constitution."
14 Notes to Change in Vibration-rate.
15 Vallery-Radot, *Precis de Pathologie Medicale*.
16 *Uruj* (ascent), *nasul* (descent), *jalal* (majesty), *jamal* (beauty), *qada* (fate), *qadr* (destiny).
17 Cf. Bechold 112, Sckade 137, Pearson and Wyllie 160 and many other authorities.
18 See *On the Diagnosis of Signs and Symptoms*.
19 See *On the Diagnosis of The Pulse*.
20 See *On the Diagnosis of Signs and Symptoms*.
21 See *On Medicine and its Topics*.
22 Many other points are noted in Part Two.
23 See *On Treating Diseases, Disorders, Obstructions, Swellings and Managing Pain*.
24 M. O. Stanton, *An Encyclopedia of Face and Form Reading*.
25 Sir A. Garrod, *The Huxley Lecture on Diathesis*.
26 See *On the Classification of Types of Disease*.
27 St. Thomas Aquinas, *Summa Contra Gentiles*, ii, 75, p. 204.
28 *Ibid*., 205.
29 See Part Two.
30 F. Hartmann, *The Life of Paracelsus and the Substance of His Teachings*.
31 See Part Three.
32 J. Bauer, Int. Med., ii, 127.
33 The essay entitled "Progress," was Gruner's Appendix.
34 See Introduction by O. Cameron Gruner on knowledge.
35 See Part Four.
36 This is the beginning of Gruner's original Introduction.
37 *Les Grands philosophes*, p. 156.
38 Ameer Ali, *The Spirit of Islam*, p. 392.
39 For instance, at Cairo, established in 684 A.H. by the daughter of the Mameluke Sultan Malik Taher.

40 Ameer Ali, *The Spirit of Islam*, p. 392.
41 *Lehrbuch der Geschichte der Medizin*, i. 662.
42 *Arabian Medicine and Its Influence on the Middle Ages*, p. 57.
43 Ameer Ali, *ibid.*, p. 517.
44 Old saying quoted by Ameer Ali, ibid, p. 125.
45 *Many Days in Morocco*, pp. 32, 61.
46 Somerset Maugham, *On a Chinese Screen.*
47 Sir Henry Howarth, *History of the Mongols.*
48 Forke, T*he World-conception of the Chinese.*
49 Others include Brucell, Wilhelm, Ging, *Das Buch der Wardlungen aus dem chinesische.*
50 See Avicenna's *Introductory Words.*
51 See Avicenna's *Introductory Words.*
52 See *On Medicine and its Topics.*
53 See *On Medicine and its Topics.*
54 See *On Medicine and its Topics.*
55 *Ibid.*
56 See *On Medicine and its Topics.*
57 J. P. Bruce, *Chu Hsi: Philosophy of Human Natur*e, p. 168.
58 Chuang Tzu, Giles translation, p. 170.
59 *Ayurveda*, 1924, i, I.; and see also Weber, *History of Indian Literature.*
60 Forke, *Chinesische Mystik*, pp. 242, 243.
61 Lancet, 1927.
62 Cf. Forke, *ibid.*
63 Hume quoted by Maher, *Psychology*, p. 238.
64 Kempis, *Imitatio Christi*, ii, II.
65 St. Thomas, *Summa Contra Gentiles*, i, 53.
66 *Gulshan-i raz*, couplet 299, p. 30.
67 *Essays in Zen Buddhism*, p. 185.
68 *Ibid.*, p. 200.
69 *Ibid.* p. 306.
70 *Rose Garden,* 1st ed., p. 120.
71 J. P. Bruce, *Chu Hsi: Philosophy of Human Nature*, i., 182.
72 The real authorship of the Libellus on the power of the hearts is disputed. Arnold of Villanova translated it into Latin (ca. 1235-1312).
73 Huineng, Susuki, *Essays in Zen Buddhism*, p. 203.
74 *Ibid.*, p. 223.
75 *Kempis, Imitatio Christi*, i., 5.
76 St. Thomas Aquinas, *Summa Theologica*, Dominican translation.
77 Ibid., liv; lv. 2; lviii. 3,4; vol. 3, p. 51-87; Pegues, *Catechism of the Summa Theologica of St. Thomas Aquinas*, p. 18.
78 F. Hartmann, *The Life of Paracelsus*, p. 217.
79 Ed. Hughes, *Lancet.*
80 Sauvage, *Catholic Encyclopedia*, xii., 313.
81 Mercier, *Manuel of Modern Scholastic Philosophy*; Logique, 1904; de Wulf, *Catholic Encyclopedia*, xii., p. 26.
82 Maher, *Psychology*, p. 520.
83 Cf. Maher, *Psychology,* pp. 35, 36; and especially Wundt, *Catholic Encyclopedia,* xii., p. 35.

84 Maher, *Psychology*, p. 9.
85 In. Met. I., lect. 2.
86 *Summa Theologica*, II-III, q. 45, art. i.e.
87 *Ibid.*, ad. 2.
88 *Ibid.*, q. 9, a. 2, ad 3.
89 St. Thomas Aquinas, *Summa Contra Gentiles*.
90 *Ibid.*, ii. 3, I. p. 5.
91 *Catechism of the Council of Trent*, 1545-1563.
92 *Summa Theologica*, especially Part I, Questions i., 32; art. I; p. 570.
93 By Lillie may be quoted from the Times, Oct. 24, 1927, p. 19.
94 See Notes.
95 St. Thomas Aqunas, *Summa Theologica*, p. 25.
96 Ibid., Inayat Khan, p. 53; Cardinal Mercier, *Manual of Modern Scholastic Philosophy,* pp. 302, 306.
97 Lecture to Notes
98 The relation between character and physique was scientifically studied by the Chinese 450 BC (cf. Wieger).
99 Cf. Wieger who is generally opposed by academic medicine; as is voiced by F. v. Muller, 1921, quoted by Kolle, Mitt. Geb. Med., 1926, 40, 371.
100 J. P. Bruce, *Chu Hsi: Philosophy of Human Nature*, i., p. 162.
101 Cf. *Paracelsus, de viribus membrorum* in F. Hartmann, p. 219. "Moreover, each individual is a member of the great organism of the world. . . "not a separate being isolated from nature" (ibid., p. 50). Individual: human world: one leucocyte: one human being.
102 *Mathnawi*, p. 169.
103 438th Arabian night.
104 See endnote 1.
105 See endnote 7.
106 See endnote 7.
107 *Ibid.*
108 *Chinese Thought*, p. 34.
109 Forke, *Chinesische Mystik*, pp. 239, 269.
110 *Description of China*, p. 104.
111 Wieger, p. 309 on Su-Wen.
112 See *On the Humours*.
113 See *On the Humours*.
114 See *On the Humours*.
115 See notes to *On Diseases, Causes and Symptoms*.
116 See *On Diagnosis, Signs and Symptoms*..
117 Ind. Med. Services.
118 *Ayurveda*, 1924, 2, i., 1.
119 Sontheimer, *Zusammengesetzte Heilmittel der Arabe*r, p. 91.
120 F. Hartmann, *Chinesische Heilmethoden*, Munch. Med. Woch., 1927; June 3rd, 935.
121 See *On Diagnosis of the Pulse*.
122 See *On Diagnosis of the Pulse*
123 The following paragraphs are interesting among many others.
124 *Arabian Medicine*, p. 34.
125 *Die Augenheilkunde des Ibn Sina*.
126 *Arabian Medicine and Its Influence on the Middle Ages*, p. 139.

127 E. G. Browne, *ibid.*, p. 26, 27.
128 *Manuel of Modern Scholastic Philosophy*.
129 Maher, *Psychology*, endnote, p. 31.
130 J. B. Bruce, *Chu Hsi and His Masters*, p. 137.

On the Breath

1 Explanatory Extension of the Subject of the Breath

Synonyms. "The breath of life" (*Gen. 2:7, Quran 32:9*); souffle de vie; ruach (Heb.); ruh (Persian, Arabic); hu (Sufi); ch'i (Chinese); prana (Hindu); [The Hindu system of physiology recognizes five breaths as supporting the body. They are: prana (the air inhaled), apana (has a downward course), samana (essential to digestion), udana (has an upward course, or passes into the head), vyana (pervades the whole body and moves in various directions, transverse and otherwise; therefore, equivalent to the "breath" of the present section.) But prana includes the rest, ordinarily speaking.-E. A. C., Kaviratna, *Chakara Sarnhita*, ii. 20]; hauch (German); Spirit (as a translation of "spiritus," for which " breath " is the better equivalent: see *On the Three Faculties*, endnote 3 and endnote 9; *spiritus* is the Latin translation of the Arabic *nafs*).

Primordial aura (J. P. Bruce, *Chu Hsi: Philosophy of Nature*, p. 101); "ether"; vivifying principle; vital fluid; vital (cosmic) force.

Definition: that which binds the vegetative and sensitive life into one connected whole. It is common to, and like in, aid living things.

"That which centers in the cardio-pulmonary center."(Baraduc, *Les Vibrations de la vitalite humaine*). "It is a subtle vapor which rises from the blood, diffuses itself to the remotest arteries, and resembles the sun in luminosity, (*Chahar maqala*, p.8)

Negative definition. "Breath" is not "respiration," "breathing," drawing in breath. Therefore it is not the equivalent of *anhelitus, nafas, anfas, Atem.*

The expression "he breathed his last" actually describes the departure of the "breath," but there are two events taking place simultaneously, and the literal respiration is only one of them.

It is not "soul" (*anima*). The latter is the Latin translation of the Arabic *ruh* in various passages.

It is not "vitality," for this is the manifestation of breath.

Vitality stands for the vegetative soul. Thus, enfeebled vitality means lessening of the ability of the vegetative soul to accomplish some or all of its instinctive drives. Therefore, it is not "life." ("Allah made life to be in breath." *1001 Nights*, Lady Burton, v., p. 422). It is not the "vital air" of the 18th century chemists. It is not even " vital drive." It is not amenable to either physical or chemical methods of investigation. It is not a force at all, and, therefore, not analogous to electricity, magnetism, heat, etc. though in the course of its activity it manifests all such phenomena.

Breath Is Not "Individuality"

Description by analogy—being immaterial, and representing a notion foreign to Western thought, breath is almost indefinable, whereas to the Eastern mind there seems little difficulty in the conception. Analogies such as to flame, a pendulum, a ladder or lift to a higher plane of being, a chain linking the three aspects of the soul to light, to vibrations, and so on, are necessarily misleading.

By picturing the breath as a sort of aura pervading the body, with a polarity correspondent with the cosmic ether (its source, whence it individualized into the human being), the conception of orientation (in time and space) becomes feasible. The angle of incidence is then to be considered, both in regard to every direction of space and to the time of day. Thus an infinite variety of constitution in these respects becomes obvious.

The substance of the breath—this is mentioned in several passages in *The Canon*. Though immaterial, the breath needs a material basis or substrate. The substance is described as twofold: (a) an aqueous vapor, in the case of healthy breath, as occurs when the humours—the source of the substance of the breath (see 1.1) are healthy; (b) a fuliginous vapor, like the mist of the early morning landscape, if the breath be unhealthy —namely because superfluities are present in the humours.

A more tangible idea of the substance of the breath is furnished by taking it as partly consisting of oxygen, for the functions of oxygen in the body are the same as those attributed to the breath which it carries. Thus to quote L. S. Beale, "Oxygen is necessary to disintegrate the soft formed material and combine with some of its constituents" (Bioplasm). That is, breath=*mf*, where *m* is oxygen.

In the Hindu system, there are ten substrates for the life-breaths, but these are anatomical (*Chakara*, i. 402).

The "primordial substance" of Chinese philosophy, the ground of all phenomena, physical and psychical, fulfills the theory of the breath. It is invisible and intangible, but manifests as matter (solid, fluid, gaseous), as psychic existence, and as spiritual existence. This substance agrees with "breath" in showing cyclical changes, passing from energy to inertia, from activity to passivity, incorporeality to corporeality. The incorporeal is "the rule of existence implanted in every living being"; and "Li" is the nature implanted by the decree This principle of activity appears in modernist philosophy as mind. (Cf. Bruce, *Chu Hsi and His Masters*, p. 109.)

The constant activity of the breath—were the breath not in constant activity, the body would be "dead." The activity consists of: (1) changes in quality; and (2) movement from place to place. Actually, both occur simultaneously, but description would be impossible without taking each form separately.

(1) Changes in quality—this is a rhythmic waxing and waning in intensity; a change from a strong phase to a weak one, and back to a strong one; a change from positive to negative; an ebb and flow; a condensation or concentration ("inspissation") and an expansion or rarefaction ("attenuation"). In the one phase, there is attraction of energy from without symbolized by inhaling air; in the other, there is repelling of energy from within symbolized by exhaling air.

These phases of movement are represented by the terms *jalal, jamal* (Persian); *jalal, jamal* (Arabic); *shiva, shakti* (Urdu); *yin, yang* (Chinese); masculine, feminine; active, passive; etc. The rise is called *uruj* in Persian terminology, and the fall, *nasul*; it is a rise from no intensity (incipience) to great intensity; there is a period of maximum intensity (maturation) and a fall from thence to no intensity (decay, defervescence, decline).

This cycle of the breath is continuous, but varies in rate hourly (every two hours), twice-daily, daily, weekly, monthly, seasonal. According to its changes, so does the feeling of well-being of the person change; according to its changes, so are there differences of bodily vigor in one and the same person. Every family, every race has its type of “breath.” Wherever we turn in living nature we can see the traces or signs of this “pulse of life”—in vegetable life, in animal life, even the greater range of human history itself; the rise and fall of nations; the rise and fall of pandemics; the solar and planetary cycles—all show the traces of this activity, though no doubt many would consider the connection with “breath” very intangible in these instances.

The explanation of this activity—this is to be found in the fact of the cyclical changes in the imponderable elements, for the two phenomena, as already suggested, are part and parcel of the same phenomenon. Thus, breath conceived as a vibration rate, is now slow, now quick; now coarse, now fine. The range and changes of vibration from “earth” (slow, coarse) to ether “ (quick, fine), and back, as has been intimated, are associated with changes of activity of the breath. These elements are, as it were, the points *d'appui* of the breath and they constitute an “immaterial” circulatory system.

Relation of breath to temperament and the emotional character—so close is the relation between “breath,” “imponderable elements,” and “temperament” that description of the one readily lends itself to being a description of one or both the others. If we trace changes in “earth,” “water,” etc., we are at the same time tracing changes in the activity of the “breath,” and we use words which apply to both “temperament” in the old sense, and emotional character as spoken of today. Dominance of “water” is as much as to say “the breath” remains in the “water” phase over a longer period of time than in other phases in this person. It also goes with “*jamal*” type of character, the exact form of manifestation varying according to other factors in the “make up,” i.e., quiet endurance, silent submission to pain, ardor of aesthetic emotion, keen sense of beauty, love of certain kinds of music, certain colors, flowers, etc. (Note, then, how intimate this idea of “constitution” becomes).

Relation of quality of breath to will power—the will power should dominate the breath. But it cannot do so consciously if the individual is ignorant of the existence of “breath.” Persons of vigorous will power will dominate it unconsciously. It would be easy to see that dominance of will power by the breath should be very common, with the corollary that actions supposed to the initiated by the personality are really quasi-automatic

Will power may be used to “develop the breath”; that is, the way the breath flows through the body, through the various (nerve) centers.

Relation to “ innate heat”–the subject of innate heat is very prominent in the pages of *The Canon*; it is closely linked with “vitality” (popular sense of the word like i.e., “enfeebled vitality,” “has very little vitality”; “full of vim). The close relation to breath is expressed by saying that as the breath wanes (*nasul* phase), the innate heat lessens; as the innate heat is restored in the course of nutritive processes, so the breath “waxes” (*uruj* phase). The rate of waxing and waning of the innate heat varies with the individual and shows a relation with the similar phases of activity of the breath. Innate heat is expended simultaneously with “breath,” and at the same time comes that indefinable phenomenon—real enough nevertheless—called “atmosphere,” “personality,” “radiance,” “aura.”

This subject bears on the theory regarding the appearance of pathological changes in the humours. Normally, the innate heat is the agent which separates normal effete matters from healthy humours. But in disease—that is, when the cycle of the breath is not in harmony with the process of formation of the humours—injurious effete matters (acrid, corrosive, etc.) appear as by-products of the abnormal humoural state, the latter being the result either of a change in the innate heat or of a conflict between this and "foreign heat" (i.e., bacterial products, see *On Diagnosis: The Signs and Symptoms*, Gruner's Introduction, "*The Guides to the Diagnosis of the State of the Patient*").

(3) Relation to metabolic changes spoken of (Lecture 2, endnote "Considered Dynamically-Change") under the picturesque title "dance of the elements." The picture of imponderable elements dipping down into the world of ponderable elements (or, to be precise, the individual human being), and entering into the changes of metabolism expressed as changes of pivot of function from C to O or H, or N, or S, or P in compound after compound, and break-down into CO_2 or H_20, etc. or as formation of tissue cells and their subsequent necrobiosis, etc.—all this is completed by the view of the breath, passing from phase to phase, from strong to weak, not merely in one organ,

(4) but in every particle of the whole being. With the ascending phase of the breath come the formation of increasingly complex substances, "generation"; with the descending phase, goes the disintegration into simpler substances, "corruption." Viewed as life-principle, we may think of the breath as controlling the vegetative faculties of the soul, which are associated by an intimate mutual relationship.

In this connection, the observation may be here noted that change of electric potential arising from the metabolism of the salts is necessary to the formation of active (as opposed to inert) fat in the body.

Hence physiological action—that is, anatomy in motion—is not merely a question of the behavior of C, H, O, N, S, P, in the various side-chains, etc. It is a sum of potentialities possessed by the separate imponderables and by their varying combinations in a particular individual at any given time. The common denominator or collective formula which represents this sum adequately is necessarily very complex, and yet it is really essential that it be elucidated before one could be said truly to grasp the real basis of a person's ill-health, or intelligently work out the fundamental bases of prognosis.

(2) The activity of movement—the second mode of activity of the breath consists of a cyclical movement, a movement in place, a movement comparable with a. circulation. During the course of this movement, the breath comes successively into relation with the several tissues and organs, one after the other until it reappears at the starting-point.

The movement may be anti-clockwise: as well as clockwise in the various parts of the body.

But there are two paradoxes here. Firstly, there is no period of time when the breath can be said to have passed a given point. It is not like an object going round and round, like an imaginary drop of blood. The breath is all through the
body all the time. It is more as if there were a series of lights in an electric circuit, and they burning the whole time, but the intensity is changing successively from point to point. The breath is always in the great centers of the body (the *chakras, prana*s but it is brightest in the liver at one moment and the brain at the next and so on, yet following a certain order. [This was realized also by the Chinese physicians as shown in the classic on the pulse (*vol. lxxx*, p. 28)].

Secondly, the circulation has no anatomical boundaries. [Possibly this idea underlies the seemingly impossible Chinese statement: the blood is inside the vessels, the spirits outside.] Not only this, but it is flowing left-sidedly or right-sidedly. This is transparently non-anatomical. Many would reject the possibility and even an attempt at proof would be unsatisfying. The justification for the statement that the breath is now left-sided now right- sided, flowing down each side separately, depends on-subtle observations which are beyond the scope proposed for this work. It will suffice to suggest just this: the peculiar attitudes adopted by all creatures (animals as well as human beings) during sleep; when standing or sitting; when exercising or at repose; also the different moods shown by a given individual—these and similar phenomena, carefully watched, furnish adequate indications of the truth of the statement. There is also a circulation along such intangible channels as the temperaments of the organs.

However, there is an actual relation to anatomical organs as well. There is no ambiguity about this. The passage of the breath from liver to brain, from heart to tissues is orderly and deliberately specified not only in *The Canon* but in the *De viribus cordis*, lest the unwary should be misled by the faulty ideas of Avicenna's predecessors and contemporaries. The heart as the center of life, and the seat of formation of the breath, is no mere fancy. To speak of the flow of the breath through the major organs awakening each center in turn (cerebral, thoracic, digestive, and genital) and then necessarily reaching the lesser organs (including the tissues and cellular elements) is to give a true picture of life. To insist also that in meeting the centers, the breath is altered; that it receives and then proceeds in that altered or renewed form to the lesser tissues, is to fulfill the great law—the law of giving and receiving; both together; simultaneous; balanced in degree. Both are true. To omit one is to speak inaccurately because one represents only in part.

Application to physiological histology—as has been suggested, physiological histology is microscopic anatomy in motion. It is the blackboard on which can be demonstrated the reality of the truths of the scholastic conceptions. So, in studying the tissues microscopically we must remember to introduce the conception of the flow of the breath through the tissue-spaces, the juice-canals, which are also the channels of the breath. Synchronous with this flow there is an attenuation of cell-substance into fluids; and a disintegration of complex chemical substances into simpler ones. At the same time, one must say the change in the breath is attenuation and aggregation of such substances.

Substances pass from the colloid to the fluid state; from the colloid to the crystalloid state: from complex to simple, and vice versa. They pass by aggregation from fluids into cell-substance (assimilation). It is all one single process. That which we see is with the aid of the microscope is the visible manifestation of cyclical changes in atom-groups, of carbon, hydrogen, oxygen, nitrogen, sulphur, phosphorus, etc. The excrescence which we cannot see on the nuclear contour of the leucocytes: for instance, is this subdominance of the several chemical elements—whether the change be the outcome of "attenuation" or of "aggregation." Not only this, but the excrescence of the nucleus is also the effect of the change in the breath which at different times belongs to different chemical elements, and so to different morphological histological appearances.

The conception of the blood-forming centers as the meeting point of two vitalities has already been suggested (*On the Four Humours*, endnote 8).

Application of the conception to pathology: (a) disease as the result of interference with the freedom of flow of breath, not only round the body, but also away from the body altogether. It is clear that an actual obstruction in a tissue (whether it can be seen with the naked eye, or felt with the hand, or whether it is in so minute a channel that the microscope is needed to demonstrate it) prevents the flow of tissue-fluids and is the forerunner of a morbid condition-a disease. But it exerts this effect primarily because the flow of the breath is obstructed and its rhythm degraded. Could the two series of events occur independently, the fact is that the former, the material of obstruction, would not suffice tog set up such a morbid condition.

The following are useful, concrete examples of diseases produced in this way. The dire effects produced by hysterectomy in young persons, once in much vogue for instance for severe dysmenorrhea; and the persistent ill-health which appears when it is done in older persons round the prime of (child-bearing) life. The explanation is to be found in the destruction of the "channels" of the breath—the severance of non-medullated nerve-fibers and even the actual removal of important nerve ganglia. This indefinable vital component of the being. which must "circulate," goes so far, and then finds a void, and its activity is turned back on itself; there is a revulsion; and the patient is aware of a great distress which nothing will (or can) relieve or jejunal ulcer following gastro-enterostomy, or excision of gastric ulcer.

(b) Disease as a result of disturbance in the rhythm of the breath. A change of rhythm, or an ataxy of the breath would suffice to initiate a loss of immunity to bacterial agents. Since there must also be an outflow of breath, any associated interference with its current would have the effect of holding back any of the isolated microorganisms which are always to be found in the tissues.

In this way the organisms would have time to develop into active colonies. Structural organic changes then appear in the body. When Paracelsus said that " life-principle may decompose and become a strong poison furnishing life to innumerable, invisible (i.e., microscopic) existences, by which infectious diseases are caused," he was not speaking foolishly (F. Hartmann, *The Life of Paracelsus*, p. I55).

(c) Loss of balance between the normal qualities of the breath and the functions of the body may initiate disease.

(d) The relation between the intracorporeal cycles of the breath and the cycles in the outer world is a factor for consideration in regard to the study of bacterial cycles in nature, outside the bodies of animals and other human beings.

(e) Sudden recovery from incurable diseases should be intelligible in view of the nature of the breath. Remembering the existence of polarity, and a point of penetration into the corporeal being, and considering the fact that in disease there is a distortion of the "shape" of the breath, it is not difficult to conceive that some outer force or power breaks through and restores the polarity to normal, in which event the sick person would be once more in proper relation to his terrestrial conditions, and be freed from the interference (analogous to the interference of light which has previously occurred in the activity of the breath. The event of such a revulsion occurring at all, whether the subsequent physical recovery be instant or only reached by gradual stages; would bring the case within the category of miraculous cure.

Changes of quality of activity of the breath are simultaneous with its movement from place to place within the body. The two aspects of the activity of the breath must be considered simultaneously, for they are not actually separate. Thus, to sum up, we picture the breath circulating from nutritive organs to those of the sensitive life, awakening as it does so the lower passions (the nutritive=appetite; the reproductive=desire (see *His Psychology*, endnote 11, "Details Regarding the Emotions"); and then the higher (the emotions, the atmosphere, the inspiration). The faculties of each organ are activated as the breath traverses them; their vitality augments, and the breath itself concurrently receives something from each center. The natural breath is the phase, then, when the breath is considered in regard to the natural or vegetative processes of the body, is located in the liver, and is associated with venous blood. The vital breath is the phase when it is located in the heart, and is associated with arterial blood. The animal (or sensitive) breath is associated with the nerve-fibers. Yet there are not three breaths, but one breath—"not three souls, but one soul." And the breath is not the "soul."

The changing activities of breath are associated with changes in the composition in regard to the cosmic elements; with changes in chemical composition. Movement of quality (type, rate, primary quality) goes with movement in regard to place.

The expressions "a matter-of-fact person," an "emotional person"; a "neurotic person," in the light of the considerations presented at such lengths are seen to be capable of interpretation in terms of corresponding types of "breath," which are dominant in the given individual (endnote 1).

All these changes have been analogized with a "dance." The breath is the controller of both aspects of the dance. It is the music of the dance which holds the dancers together. When the music ceases the dance ceases, or degrades into a meaningless disorder. And the ceasing of the dance is "death"; and the degradation is the subsequent decomposition processes.

The player of the music, and the movements of the two dancers should blend harmoniously to make the perfect dance. What if there be inattention on the player's part? What if he should not correspond to the capacities and capabilities of the dancers? What if the giving and receiving between the music and the dancers should fail at any moment? Surely, then there is disease. Whatever modern medicine has to say about etiology, this fact remains at the root of the phenomena of all disease. In health, the dancers depend on the player, and their dance is so perfect that they always respond to his tune.

But there comes the time when the (hidden!) Improvisor of the music cries out "Halt!"

The following repetition of some of the important facts so far discussed is justifiable for still greater precision.

Abbreviations: a, animal, b, breath; B, body as a whole, C, vital centers (heart, liver, brain, gonad); f, faculty; h, heart; j, vegetative; l, "life"; L, life-principle; m, mind; n, natural; r, rational; s, sensitive or sentient, or sensuous; S, soul in the Platonic sense; sp., spirit, v, vital.

(A) General Statements :_

L exhibits *jf, sf, rf,* and *vf.*

But *L* is not the same as *jf, sf, rf,* and *vf*; or the same as *(j.s.)l.*

L is not = *jf* + *sf* + *rf* + *vf*

L is not the same as *S.*

S is not the same as *L*; or *m*; or *sp.*

S includes *L, b, jl, sl, rl, vf.*

b is not *l*, or *L*, though almost equivalent to *l*.
l implies *b*.
af (Avicenna) belongs within the domain of *sf* and *rf* (scholastic).
jl (scholastic) comprises *vf* and *nf* together (Avicenna).
sl (scholastic) comprises *vf, nf,* and some *af* (Avicenna).
sl (scholastic) is equivalent to *nf, vf, (af-rf)* (Avicenna).
rl (scholastic) comprises *vf, nf, a*f (Avicenna).
rl (scholastic) includes *jl* and *sl* (scholastic).

(B) Special Statements

(i) The three chief views of the nature of a "person" are:

Modernists or scientific or rational	*B+m*
Popular or Platonic	*S* and *B* or *S + B*,
Aristotelian	*S.B.*, or *S x B*

(ii) The scholastic view may be thus expressed -

"Nature" is *L.B.*; the "vegetable nature" is *jl.B*; the "animal nature" is *jl. sl. B;* "human nature" is *jl. sl. rl. B.*

(iii) Comparing the description given by Avicenna, with that given by St. Thomas, we have:

Avicenna	*(b, nf, af*), B (C)
St. Thomas	*L.B.*; or (*jl, sl, rl*) B

2 It may be noted that corporeal bodies receive life when they enter into the composition of living matter, whether of protozoa or the like, or of highly organized animals and lants. The author does not say that all corporeal bodies are "forms of life," as some have assumed. The distinction between matter and form already discussed (see *On the Elements*, endnote "*Explanatioory Extension of Lecture 2: On the Elements*") makes clear that which is expressed slightly differently in the preceding passage. It should be borne in mind that the first principles are really neither "matter" nor "form;" the discussion in the text is relevant only because the listener is supposed to have failed to realize this. Although the first-principles are co-terminous with the "infinity" of the universe, they have not either mass or volume. The comparison between a "point" and a "world" is characteristically medieval.

3 Differences Between Potentiality and Disposition

Potentiality	*Disposition*
1. Pertains to equally both contraries.	Does not.
2. One and the same person can be glad and sad.	Optimism and pessimism can only exist in distinct persons
3. Is perfected into a disposition.	Is perfection of potentiality towards one or other contrary.
4. To pass one's life with a breath of sad or potentiality is one thing.	To pass one's life with a breath of sad or glad disposition is another.
5. Glad or sad potentiality can harmonize.	Glad or sad disposition does not.

Potentiality	*Disposition*
6. Potentiality for both contraries is inseparably inherent in the breath from the very first.	Disposition towards a contrary (emotion) is not inseparably inherent in the breath from the outset may appear under the influence of supervening agents.

4 'Delight is a perfection of operation," *Summa Contra Gentiles*, xc, p. 190;; "joy and delight differ in aspect. For delight is caused by a good conjoined in reality, while joy does not require this conjunction because the mere repose of the will in the thing willed suffices for the notion of joy. Therefore, delight is only in a conjoined good if it be taken in its proper sense whereas joy is in a separate good" (*ibid*, p. 191).

5 Cf. *The Theory of Pain*.

6 This passage is characteristically Sufic. The reference being to the effect of purification of the "breath" in the exercises culminating in "*shah hal*"; the personal success and accuracy of the physician in his dealing with the sick being progressively enhanced the more the purification of his "breath" is secured. The rarefaction of the breath, and the replacement of coarseness by fineness are desirable in all, but come from experience and not from study.

7 Disposition of Mind and Corresponding Character of Breath

Disposition of Mind	*Corresponding Character of Breath*	*When Met With*
Cheerful	Quantity: plentiful Temperament: balanced Substance of breath: brilliant, full of light	
Gloomy	Quantity: scanty	In convalescence In prolonged illness In old age
	Temperament: unbalanced	In disease
	Substance: dense and gross	In old age; melancholy
	Substance: attenuated	In women during convalescence
	Substance: confused	In melancholy

8 Compare the following: "all the passions of the irascible appetite rise from the passions of the concupiscible appetite and terminate in them; for instance, anger rises from sadness, and having wrought vengeance, terminates in joy," (St. Thomas Aquinas, *Summa Theologica*, Dominican translation, 81, a. 2; p. 130).

9 Cf *Ps*. 118:32; 2 *Cor*. 6:11.

10 Relations Between the Various Blood-states and the Several Emotions

Blood	*Effect on Breath*	*Effect on Emotional State*
Plentiful, bright, hot	Oxidative process active; movement swift.	Tendency to anger.
Plentiful, bright, attempered	Abundance of clear breath of laudable substance and attempered.	Tendency to delight.
Bright, watery, cool, tenuous	Oxidative processes slow; breath heavy; moves centrifugally; less is formed; more is dispersed.	Tendency to fear; neither joy nor anger; heart tends to be weak.
Thick, turbid, over hot	Breath turbid as the blood tends to "inflame," the breath thickens, and fails to cool properly.	Tendency to sadness and even continual vexation. Therefore emotion persists.
Rarefied; bilious humour increased	Breath of intense heat and rarefied.	Anger which comes and goes.
Ditto but also bright and clear		Joy.
Thick but not turbid (rarely met with)	Thick but not turbid.	Not sad but strong and bold. Very little anger because joy neutralizes this.*
Thick, not turbid, cold	Thick, cold, not turbid.	Timid, dull, upright.
Thick, turbid, cold		Gloomy, solitary; a person of rancor and resentment; anger arises only at great provocation.**

* Joy easily overcomes the emotion of anger. It is sadness that fosters anger because anger is an impulse to expel. Happy things harmonize with pleasure and pleasure entails a tendency to attract or gather in. Therefore, it will need a bid thing to make such a person angry; and as a very concentrated breath will result, there can be very little fear.
** The anger will not last as long as it would in hot-blooded people (in whom other like conditions are associated), but longer than it does in persons whose blood is rarefied. Therefore, he comes to be a man of resentment, because the disposition to hate implies the persistence of hurtful images in the imagination.

Notes

Notes

Notes

Notes

www.ingramcontent.com/pod-product-compliance
Lightning Source LLC
LaVergne TN
LVHW040331141225
827532LV00001B/104